The BIG BOOK Series of Reminiscing –

FRIENDLY DOGS & ROLLING RIVERS

A Collection of Pictures
For Our Loved Elders

ISBN: 9798387226670

Created by Lauren C. Reynolds

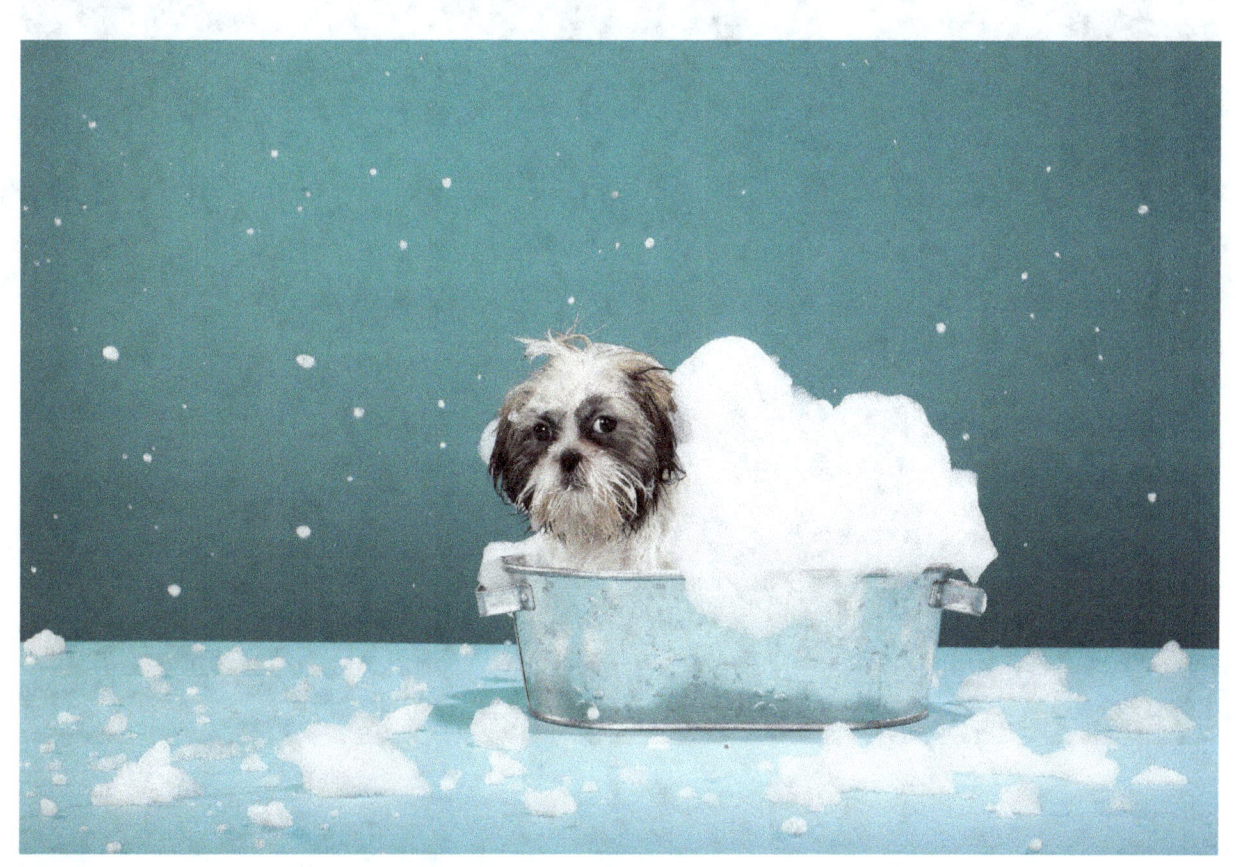

Bubble Bubble....

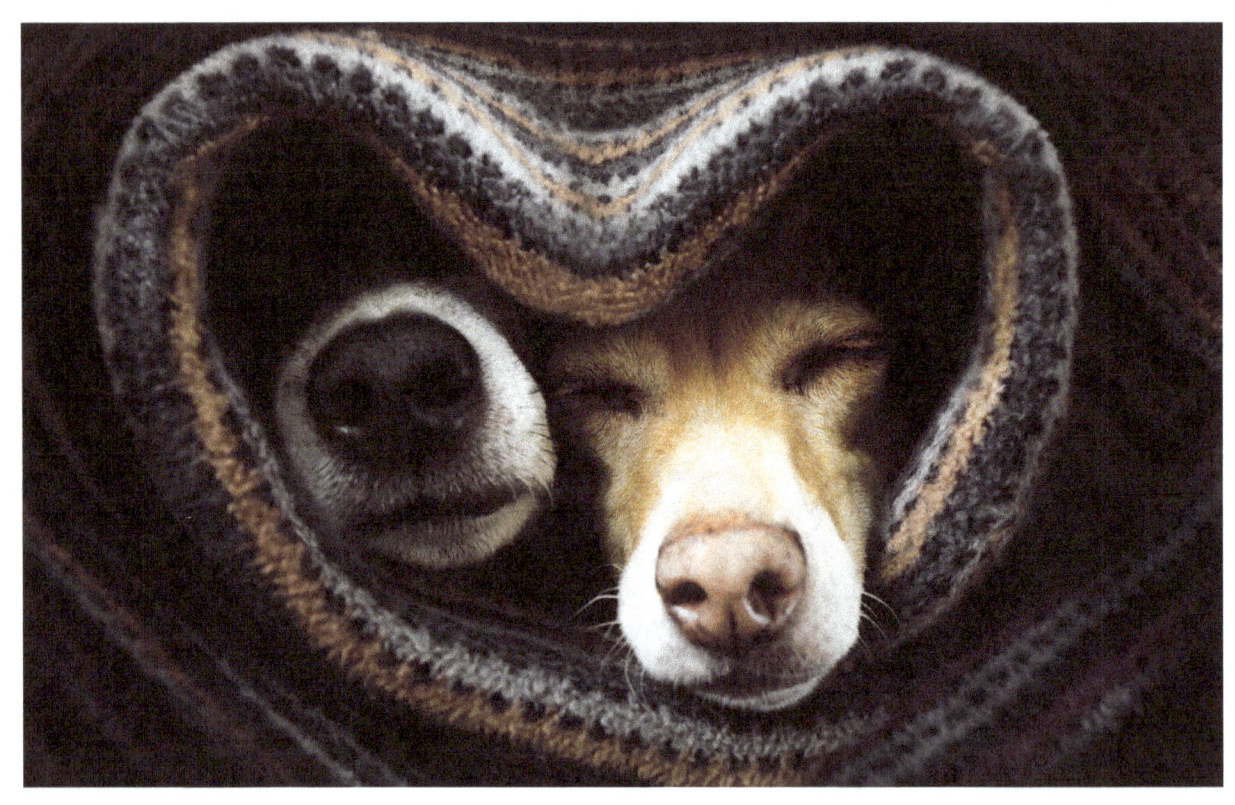

Snug as a bug
.........in a rug

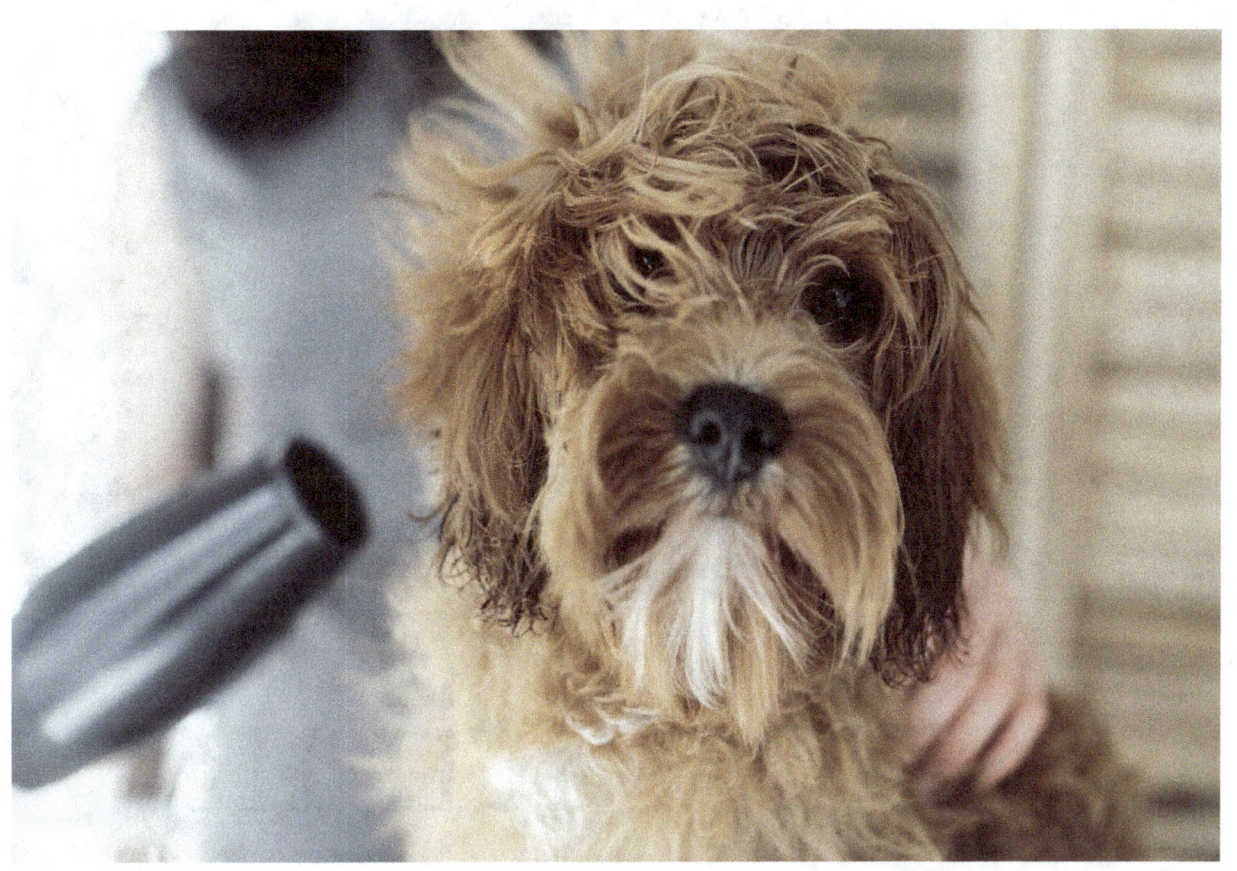

Messy hair

Don't care

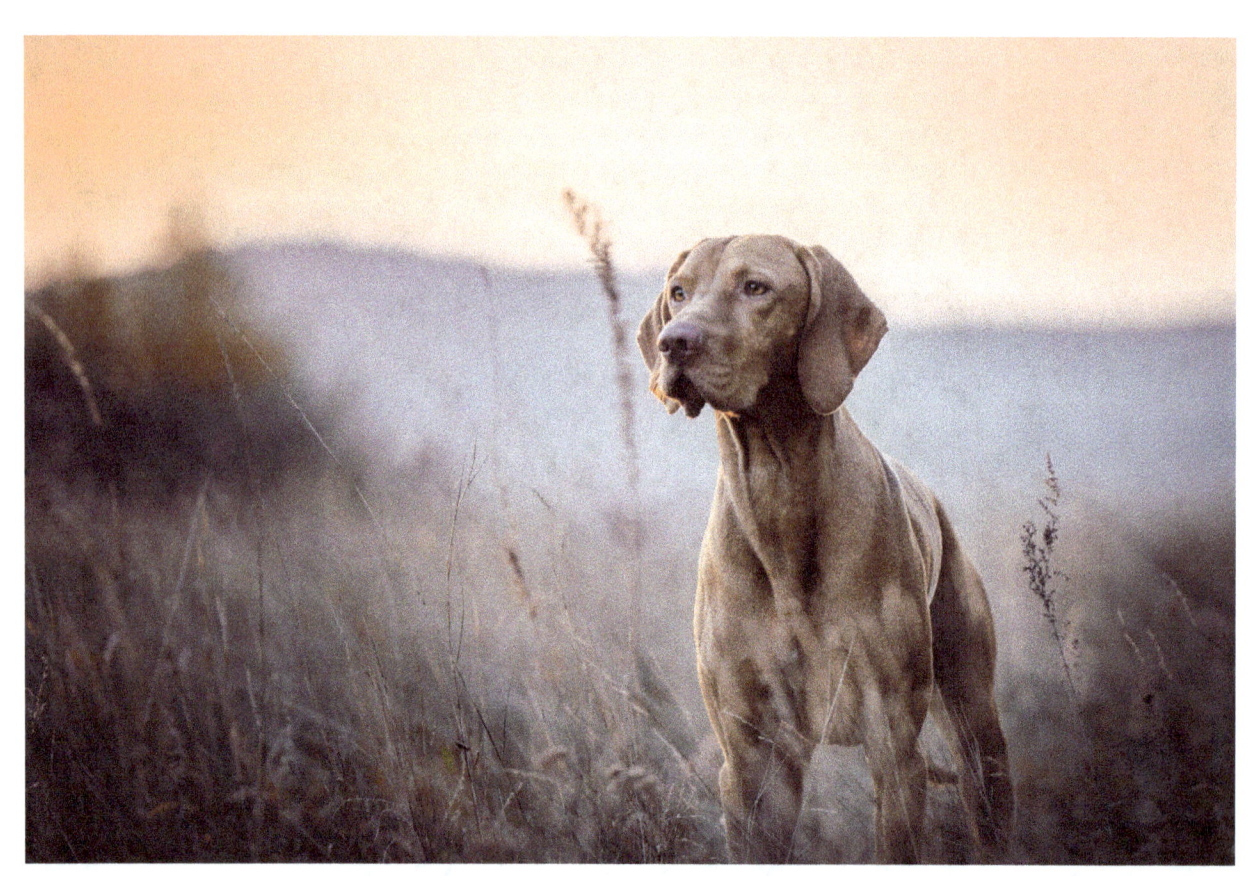

I spy with my
eye

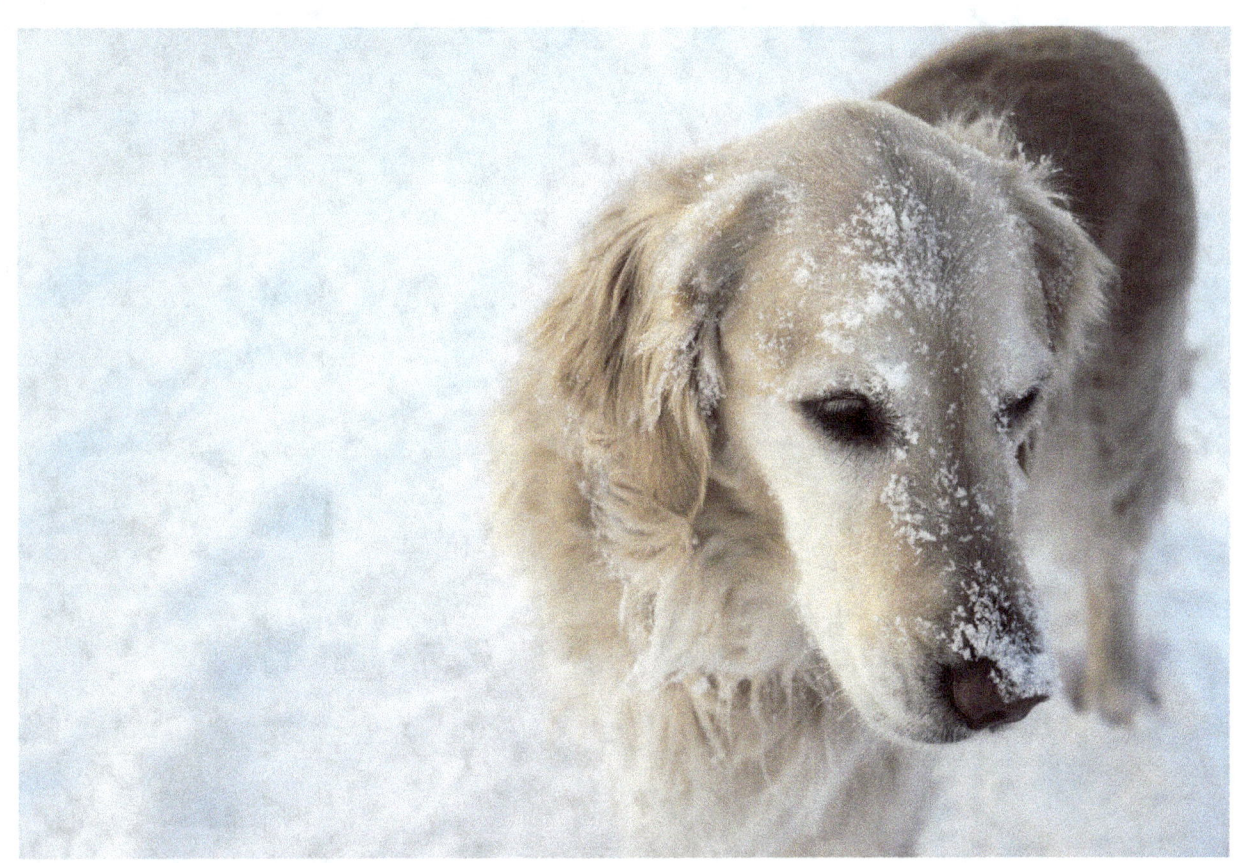

I am a special
snowflake

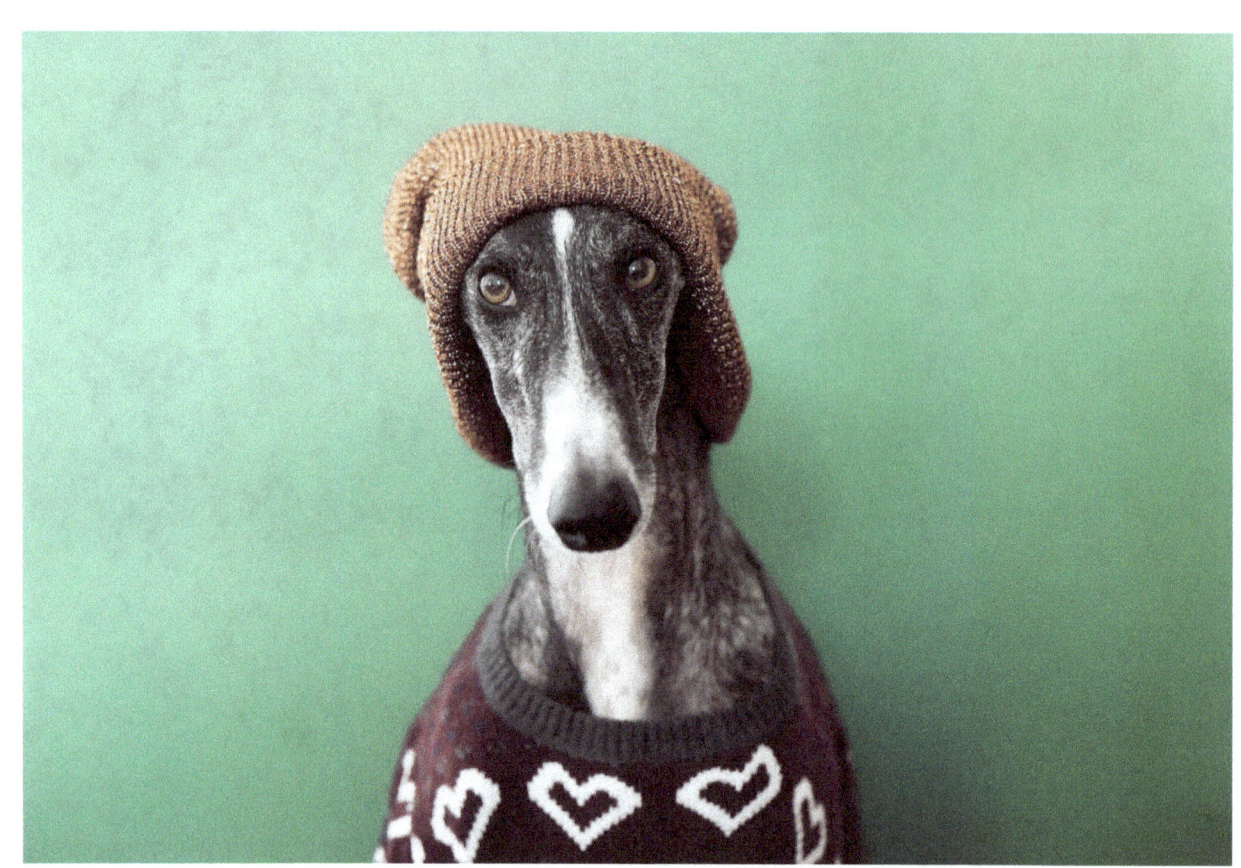

Sweater
weather

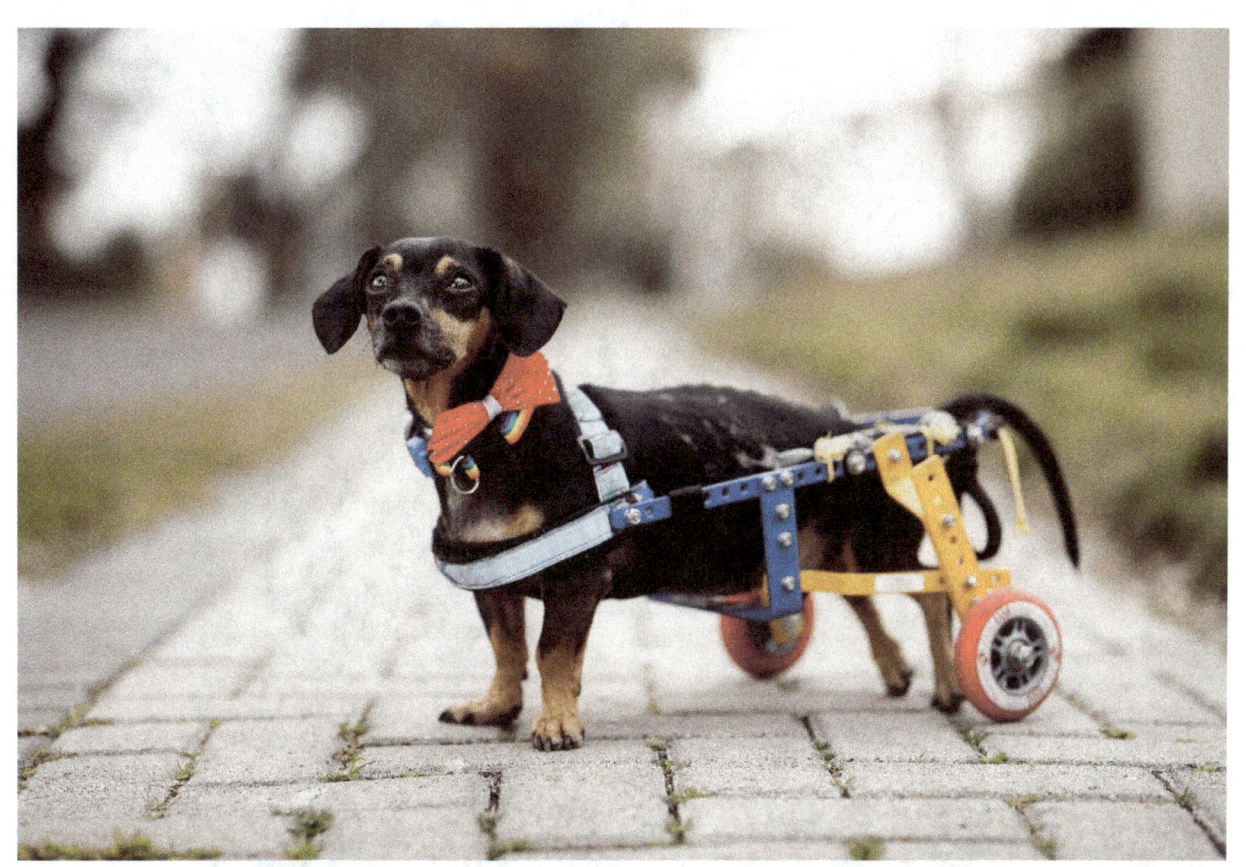

I can do anything!

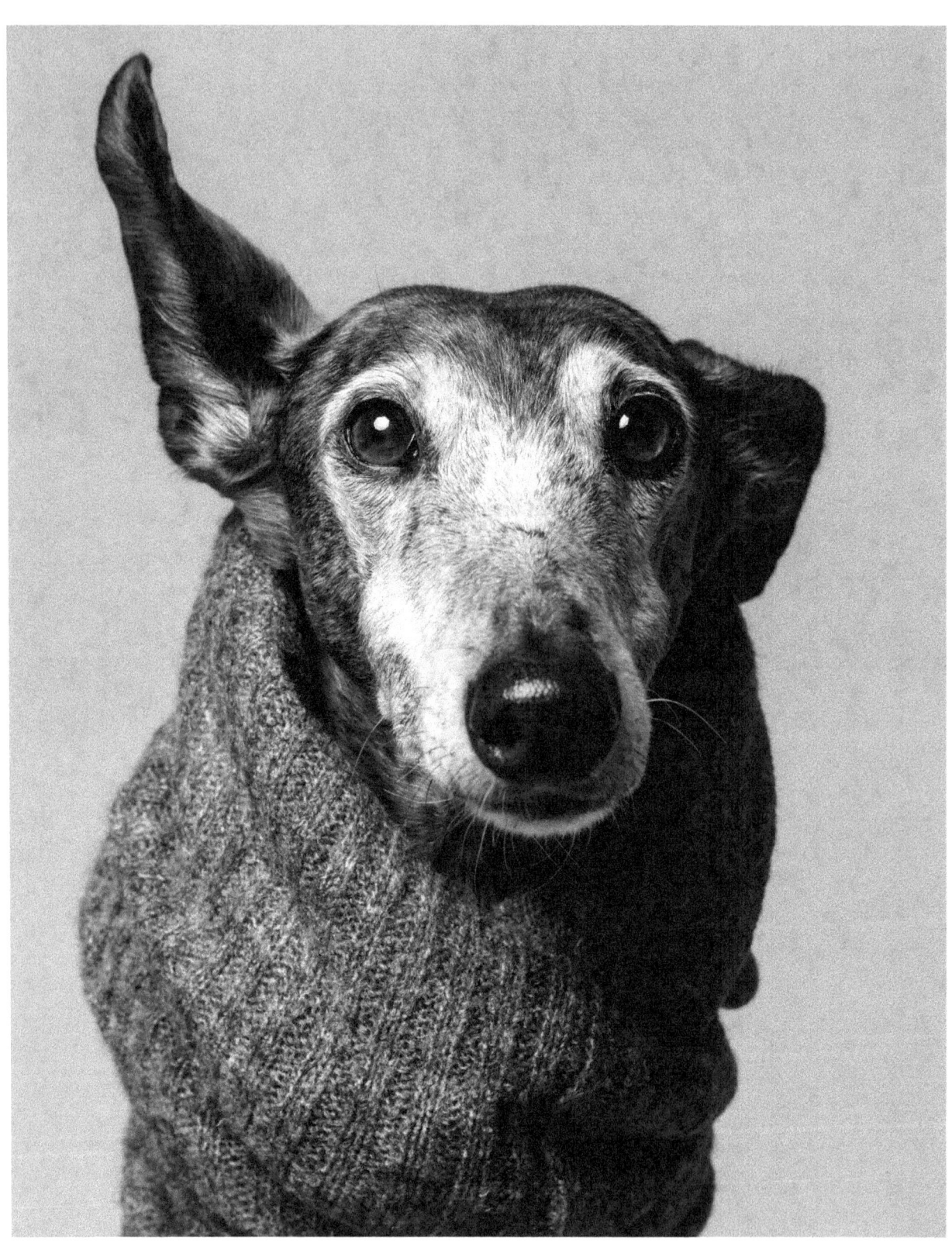

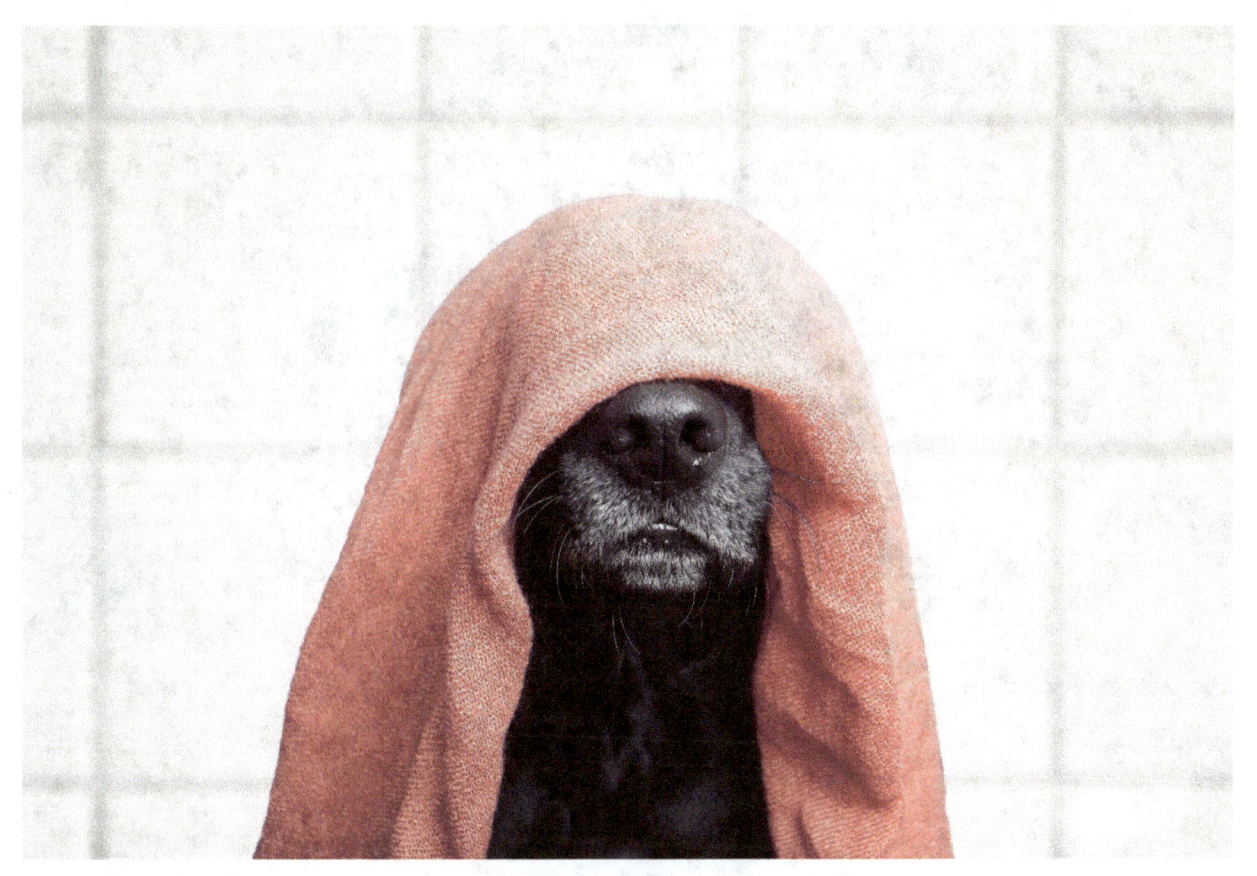

Peek A

Boo

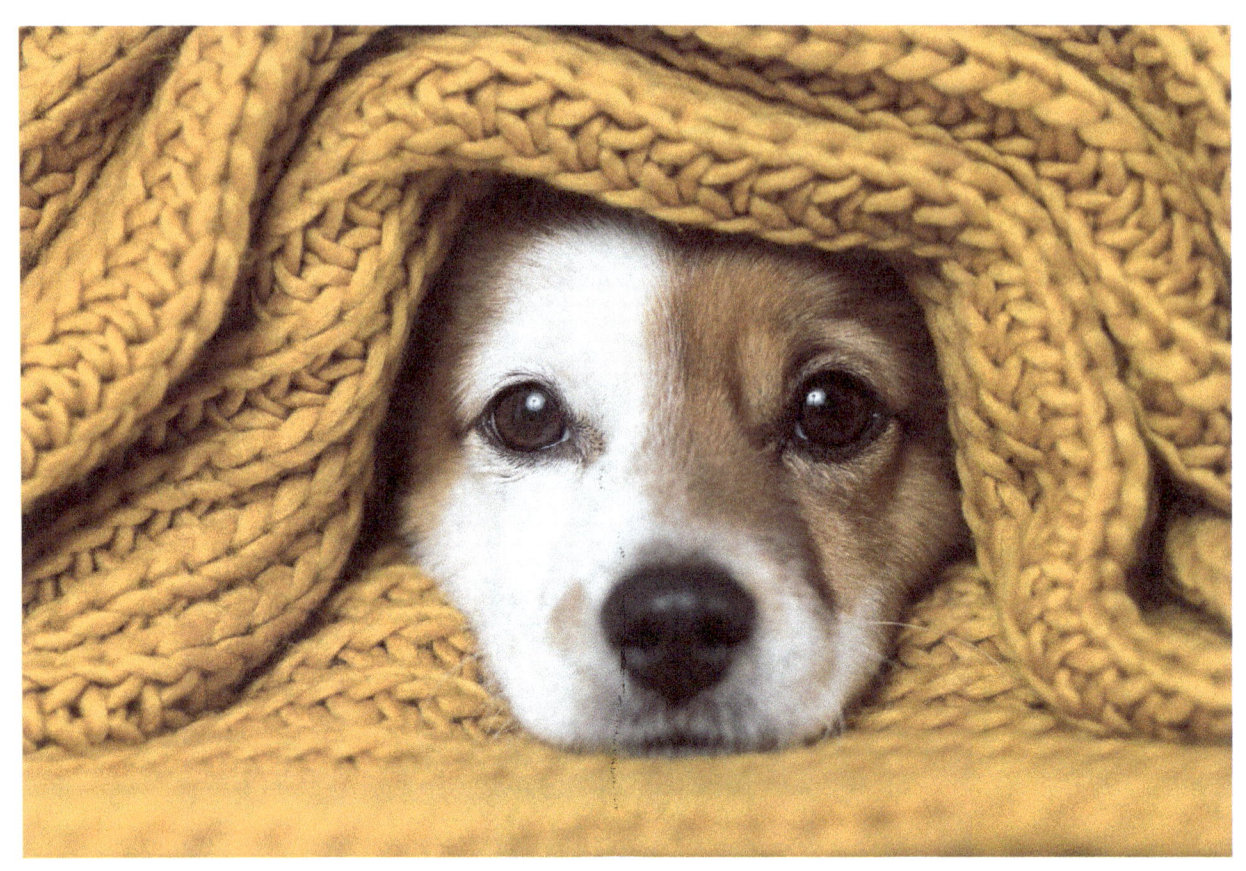

Snuggle
time

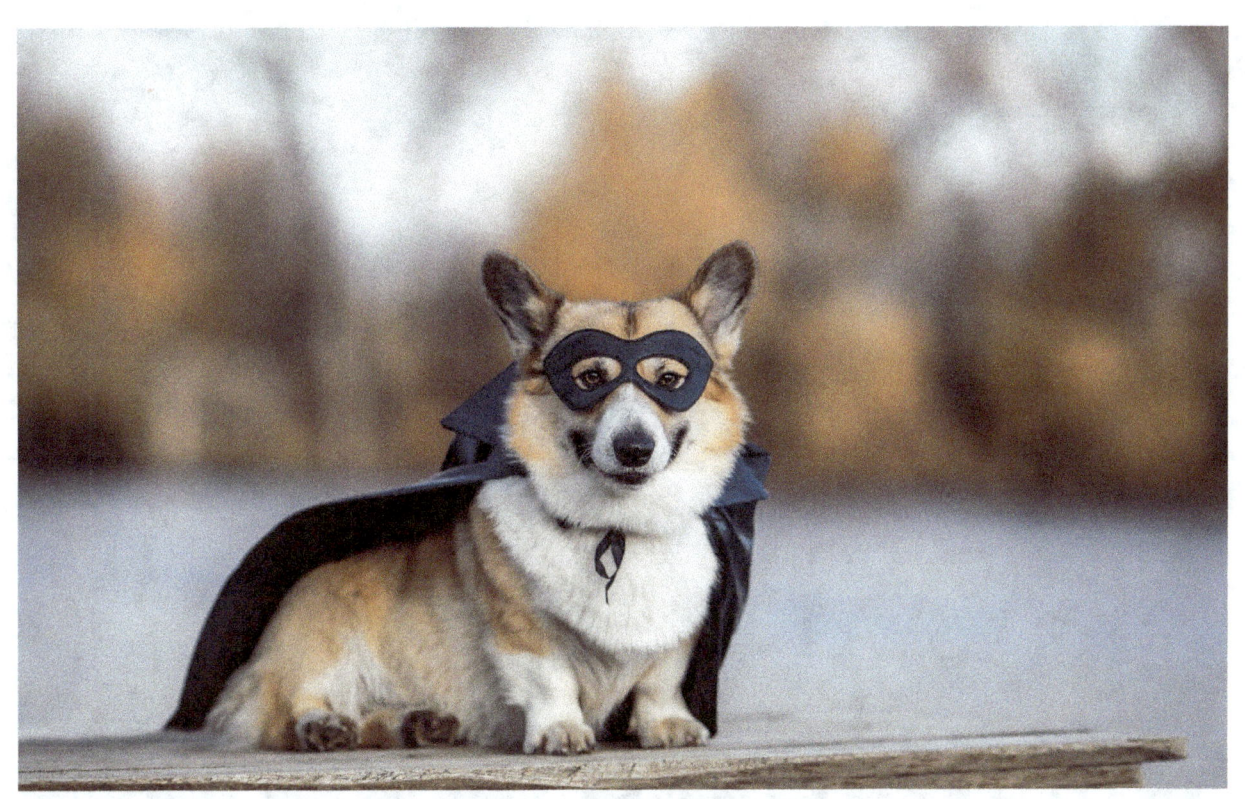

Super
Corgi!

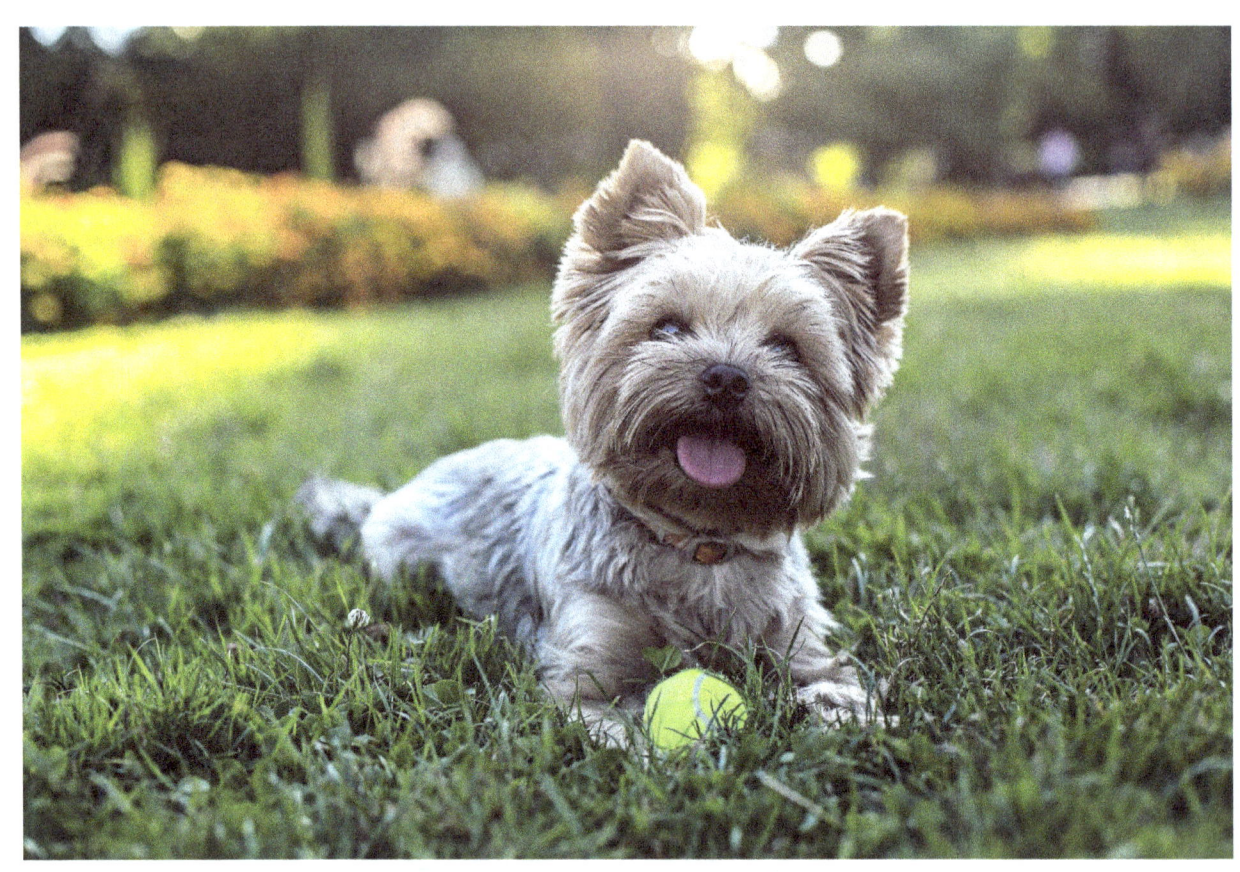

I love my Ball!

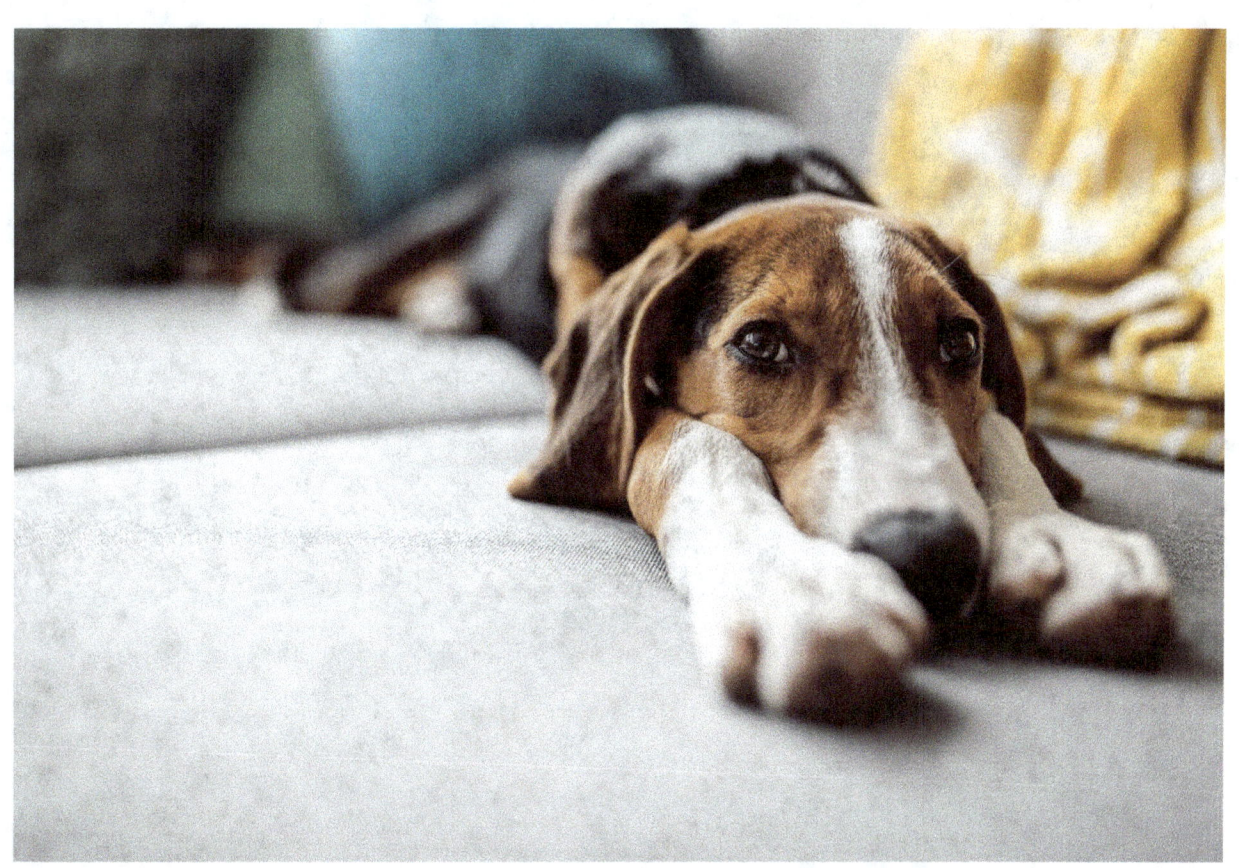

Stretch!

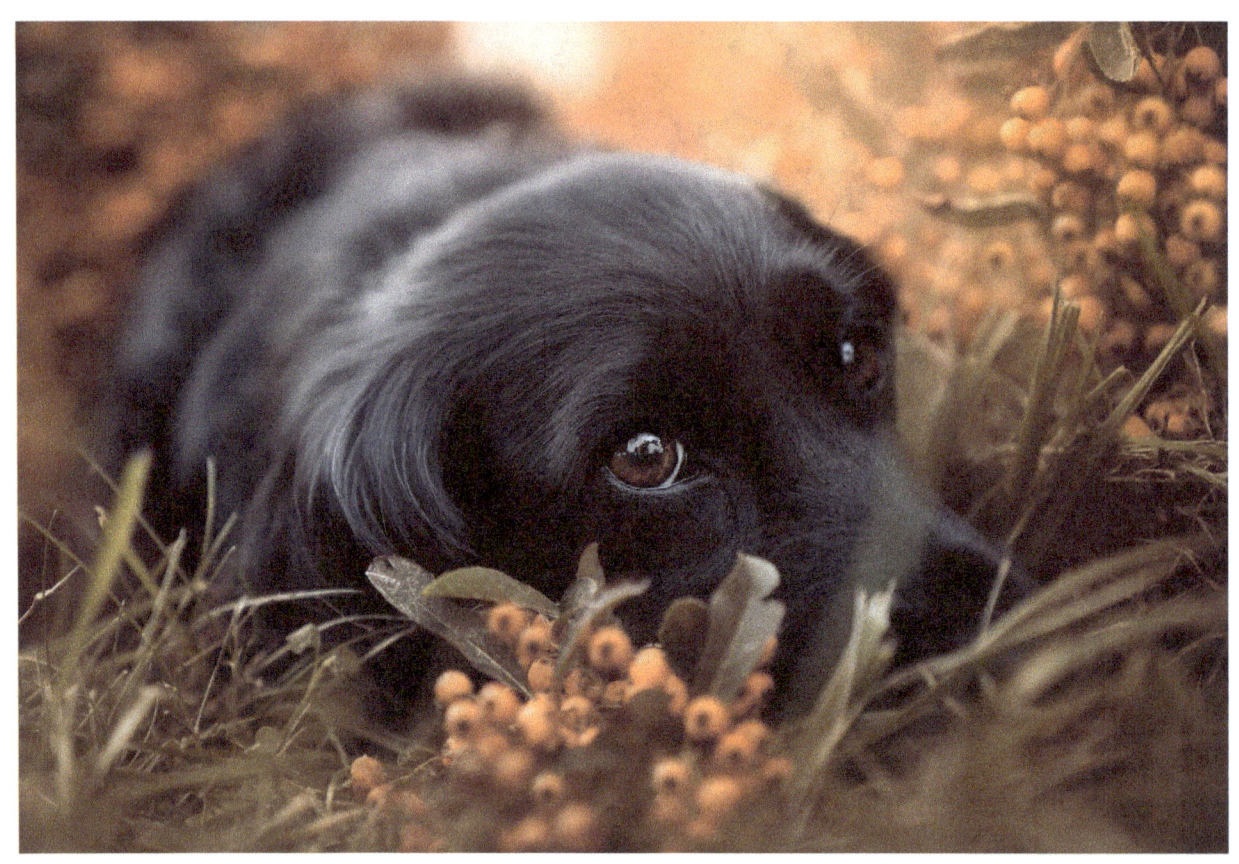

Shy Sweetie

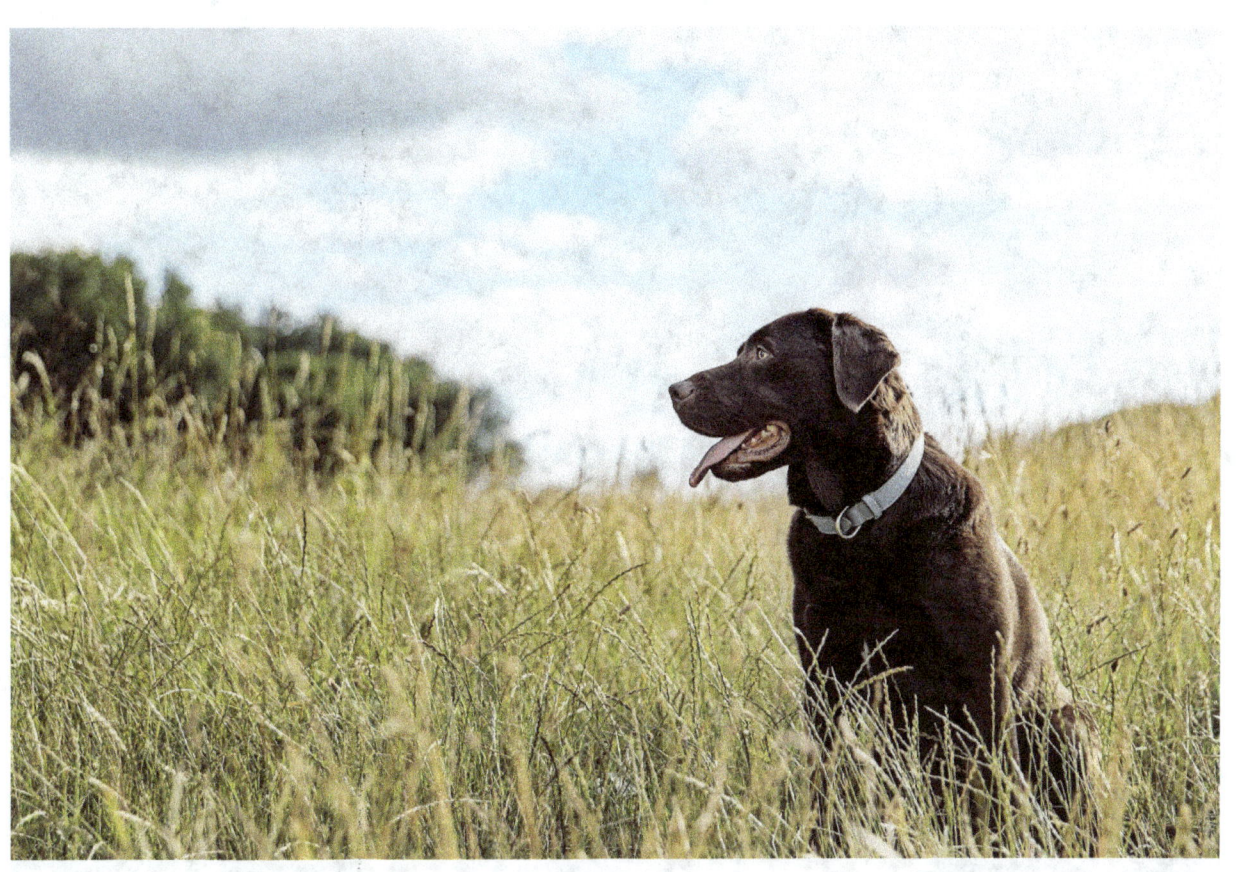

Let's Explore
Together

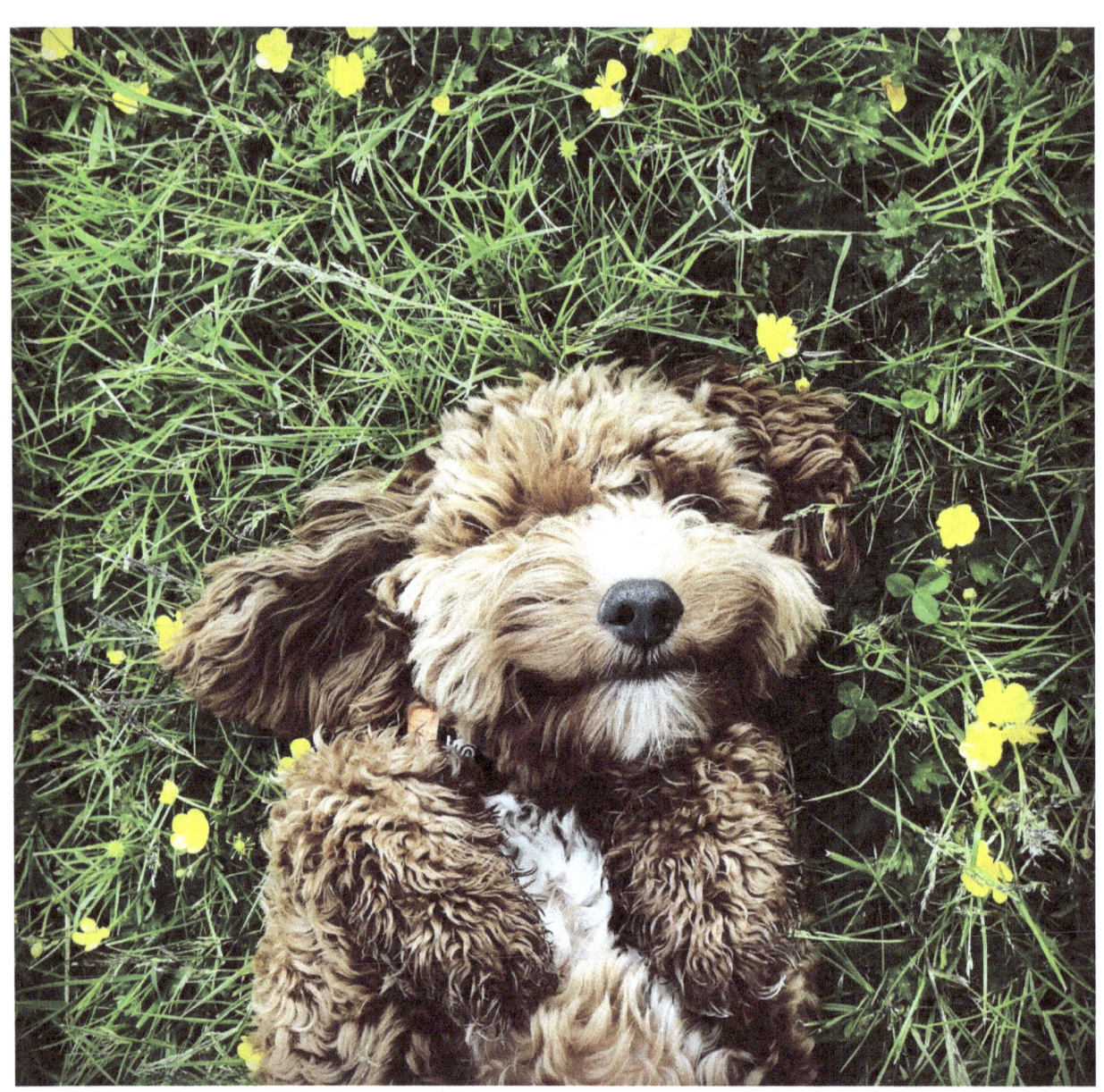

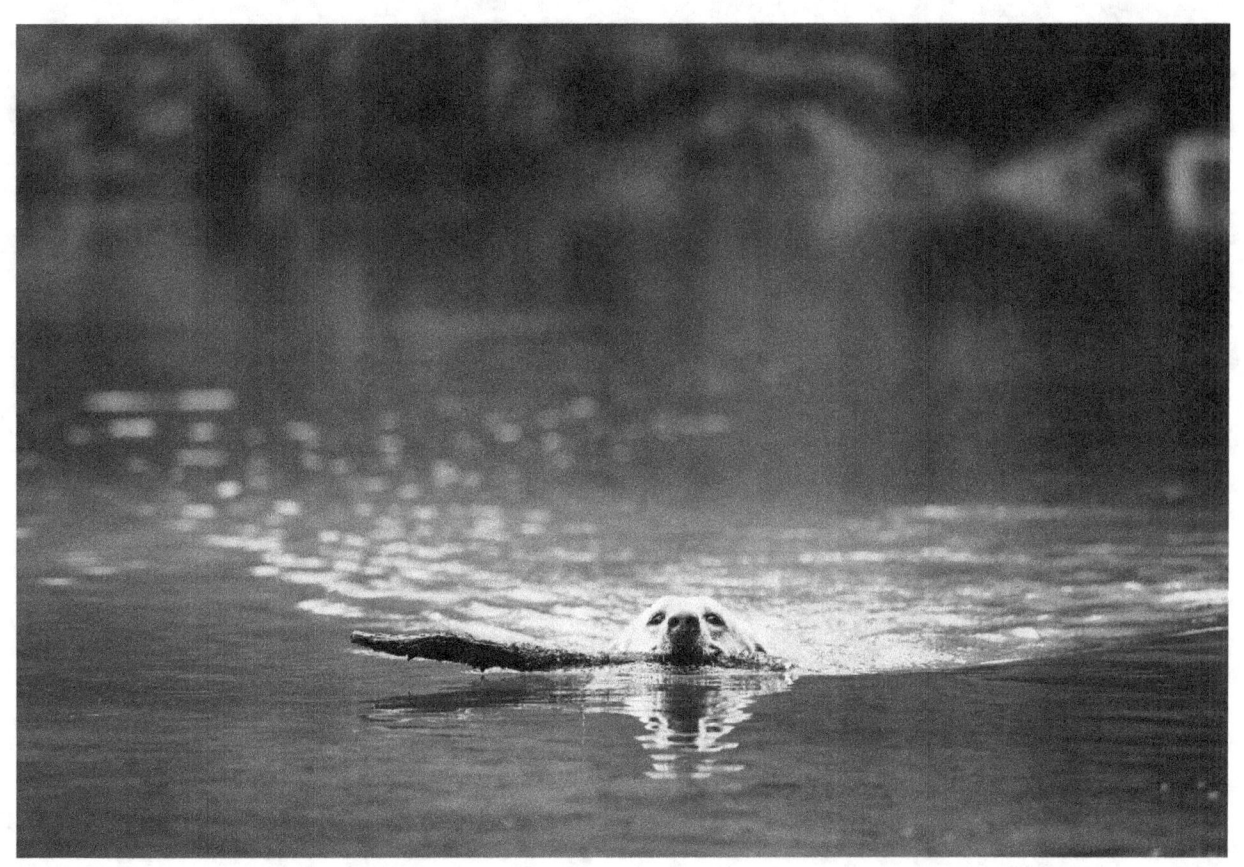

A Good Swim

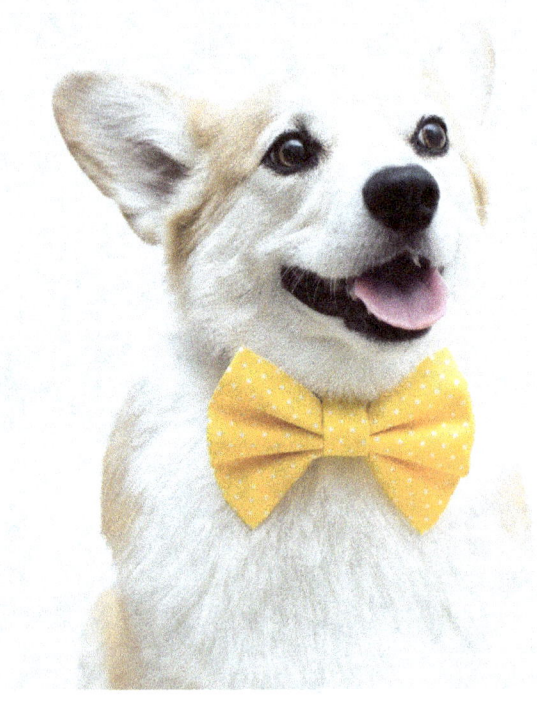

I'm all dressed up!

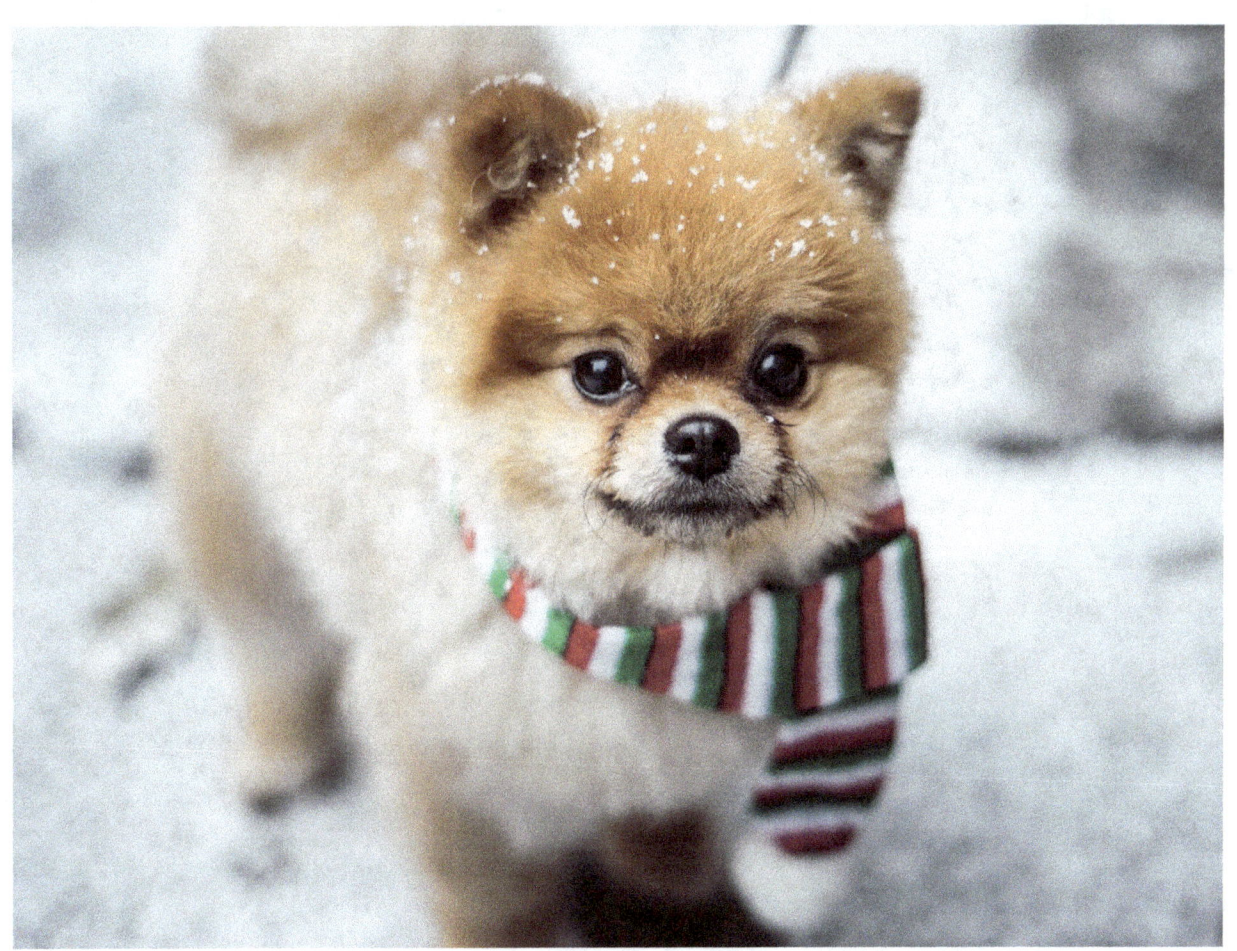

Brrrrrrrrrrr

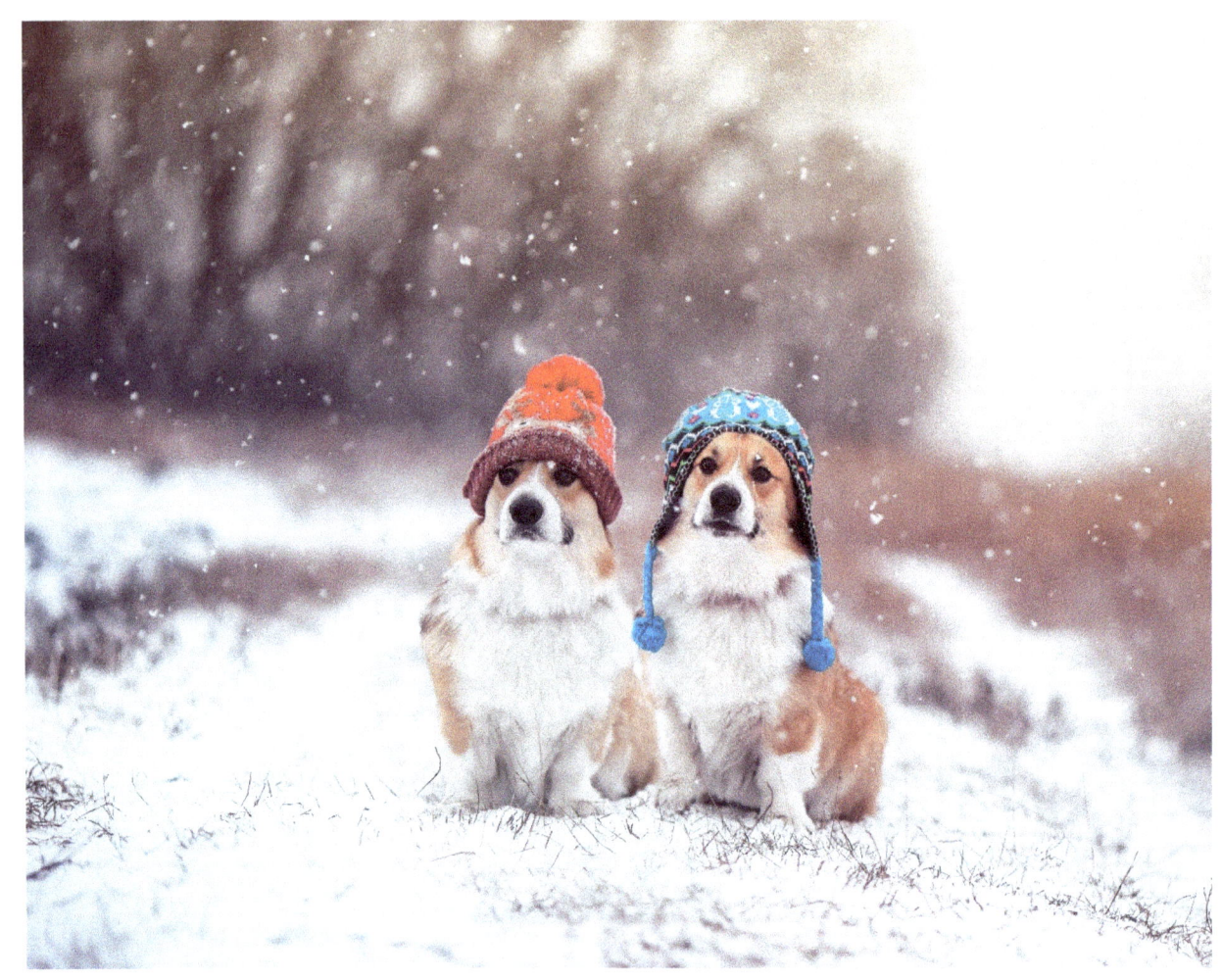

Best friends

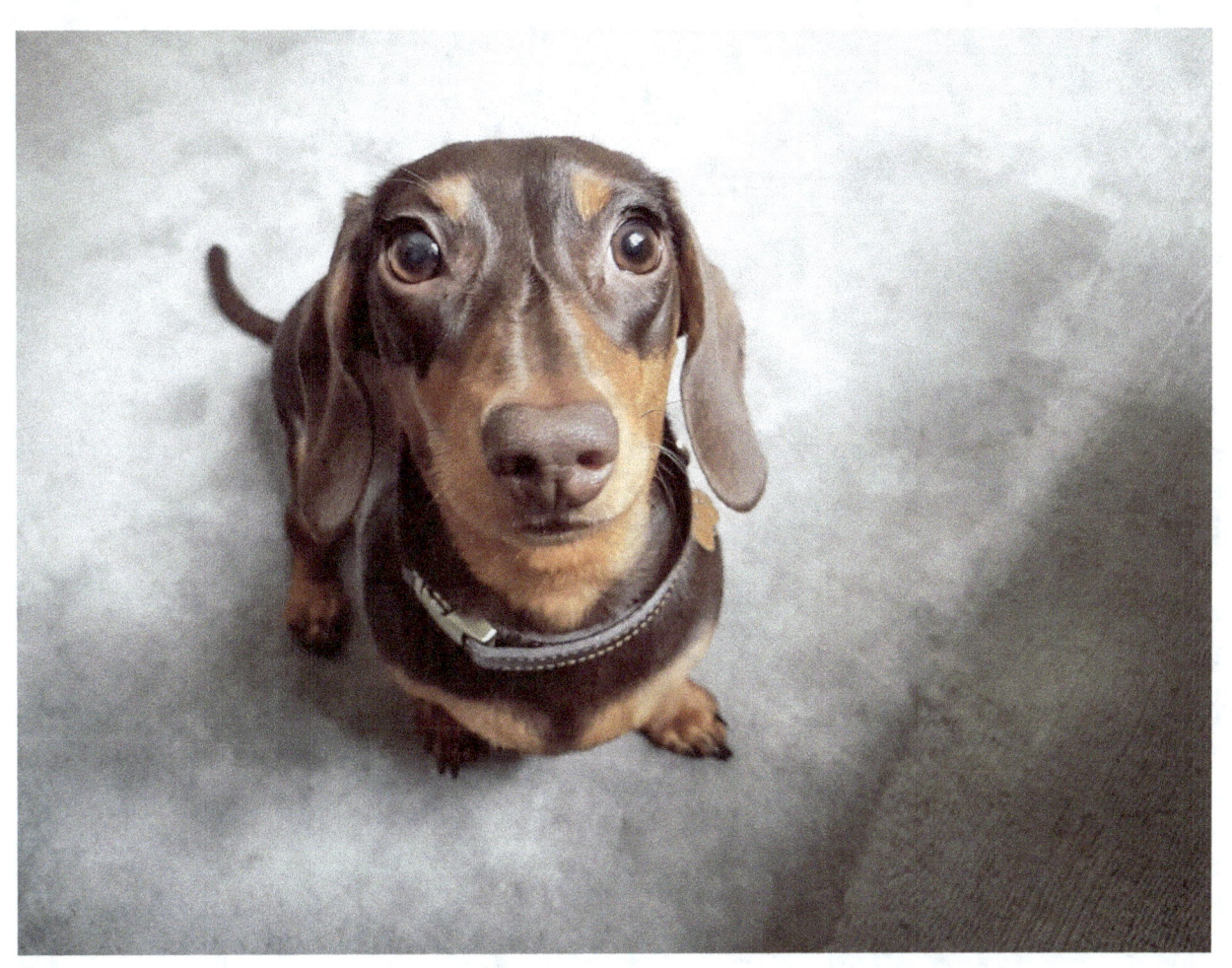

Waiting
eagerly

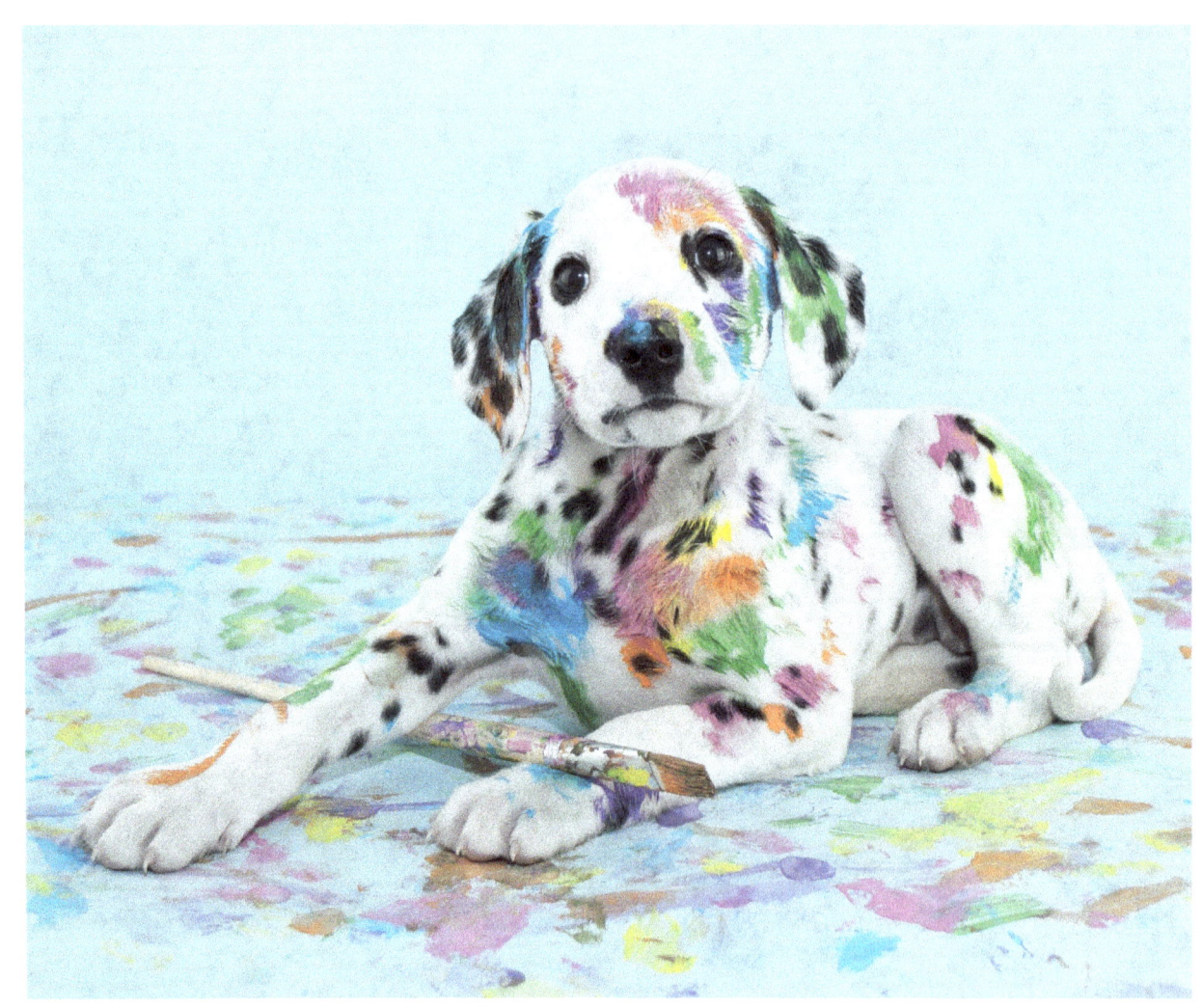

I painted a
rainbow

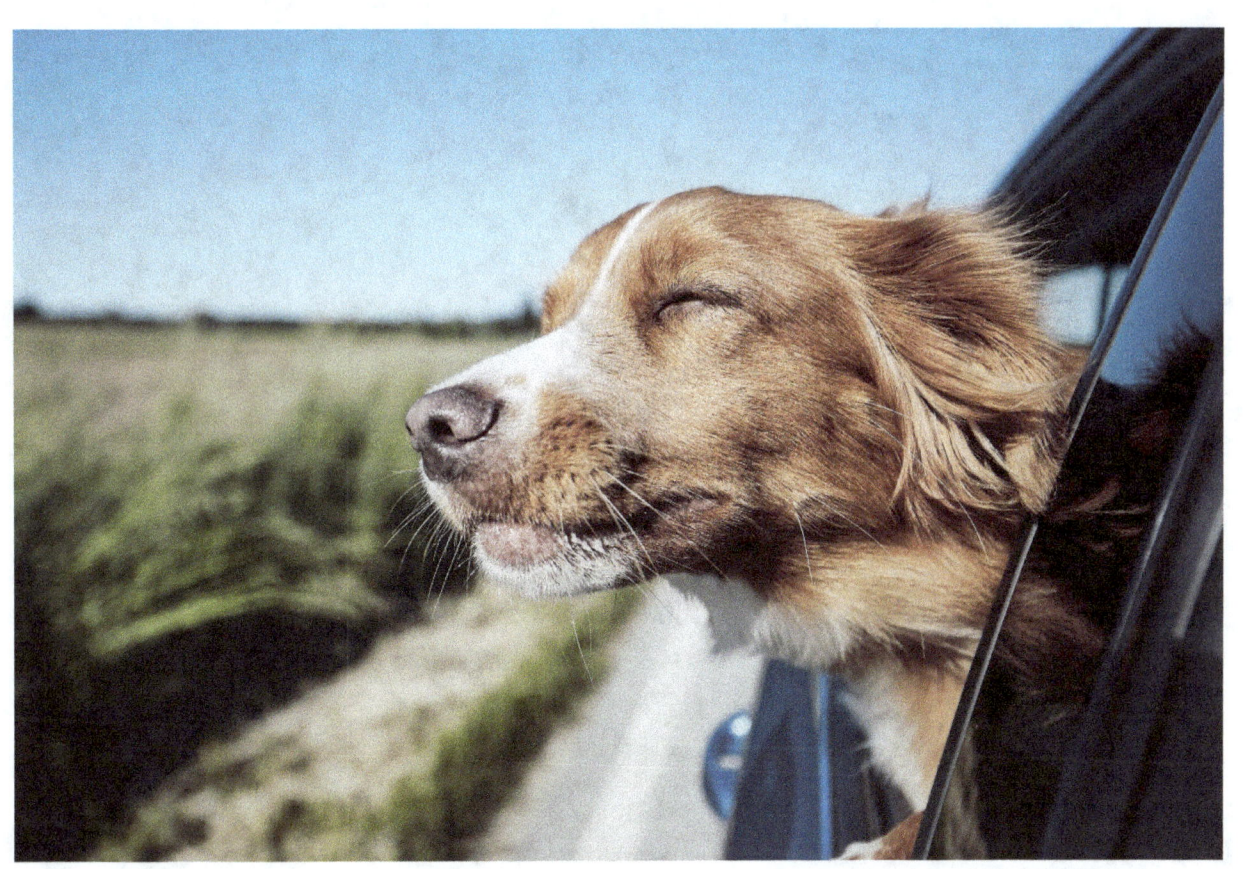

Free and easy

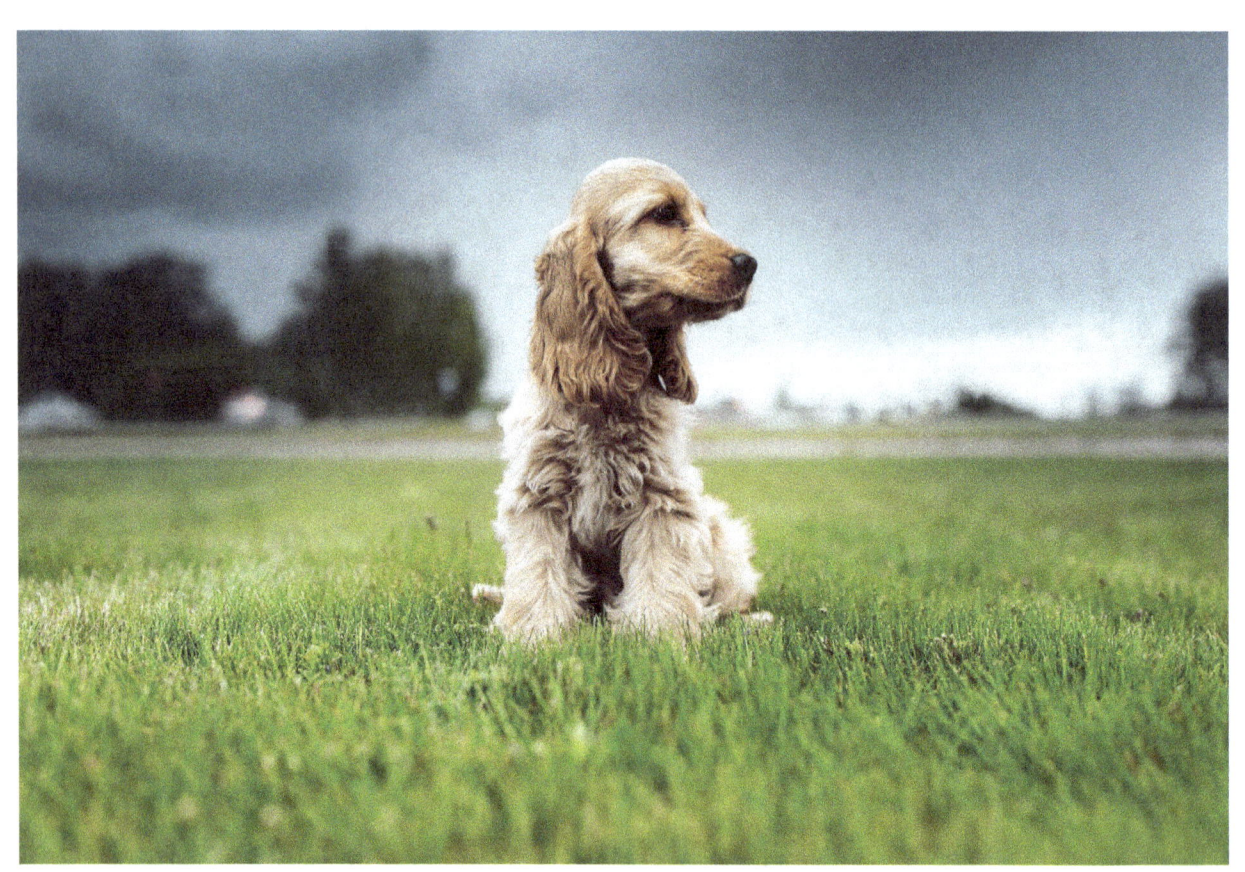

Do you think it will rain?

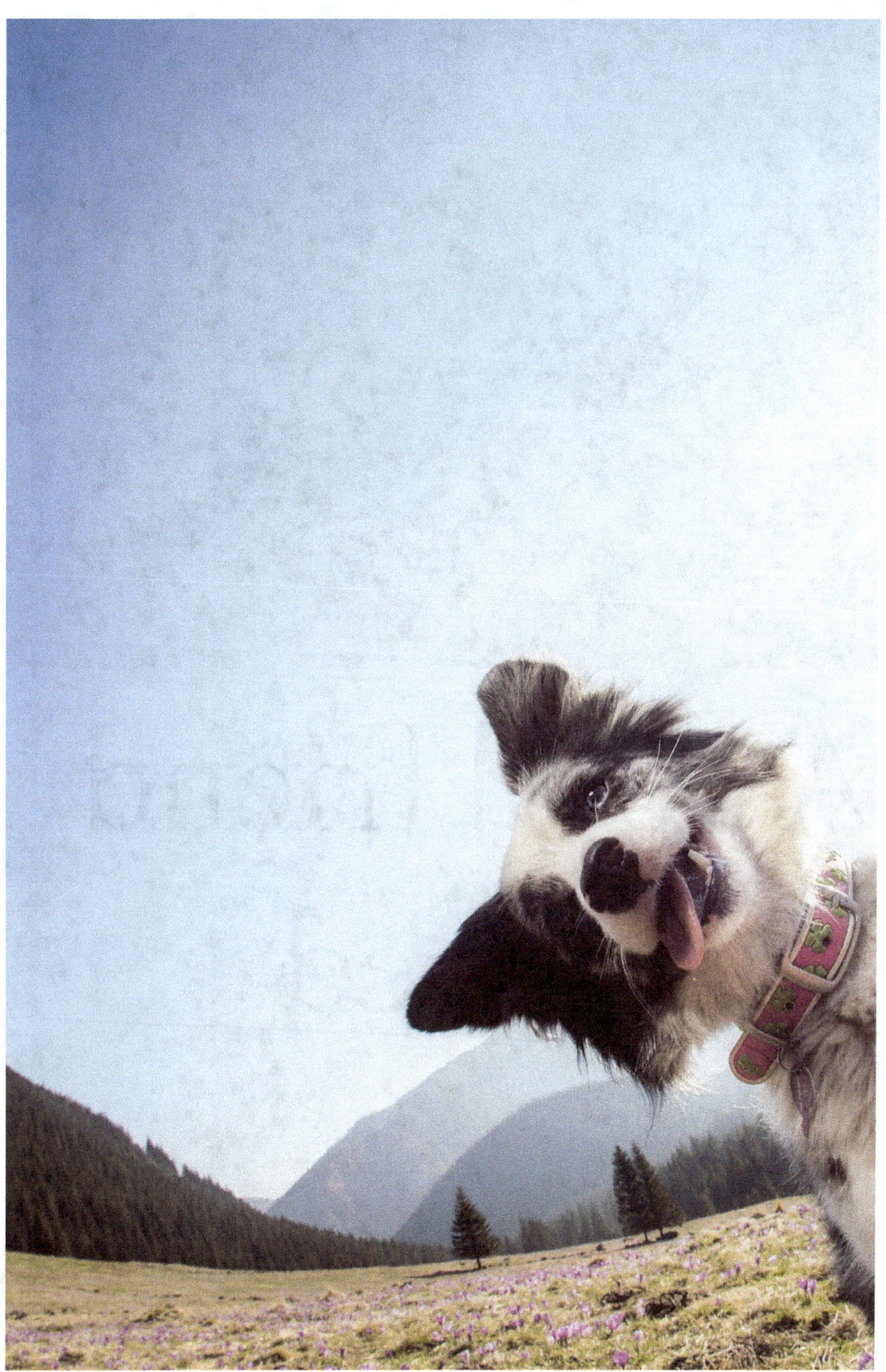

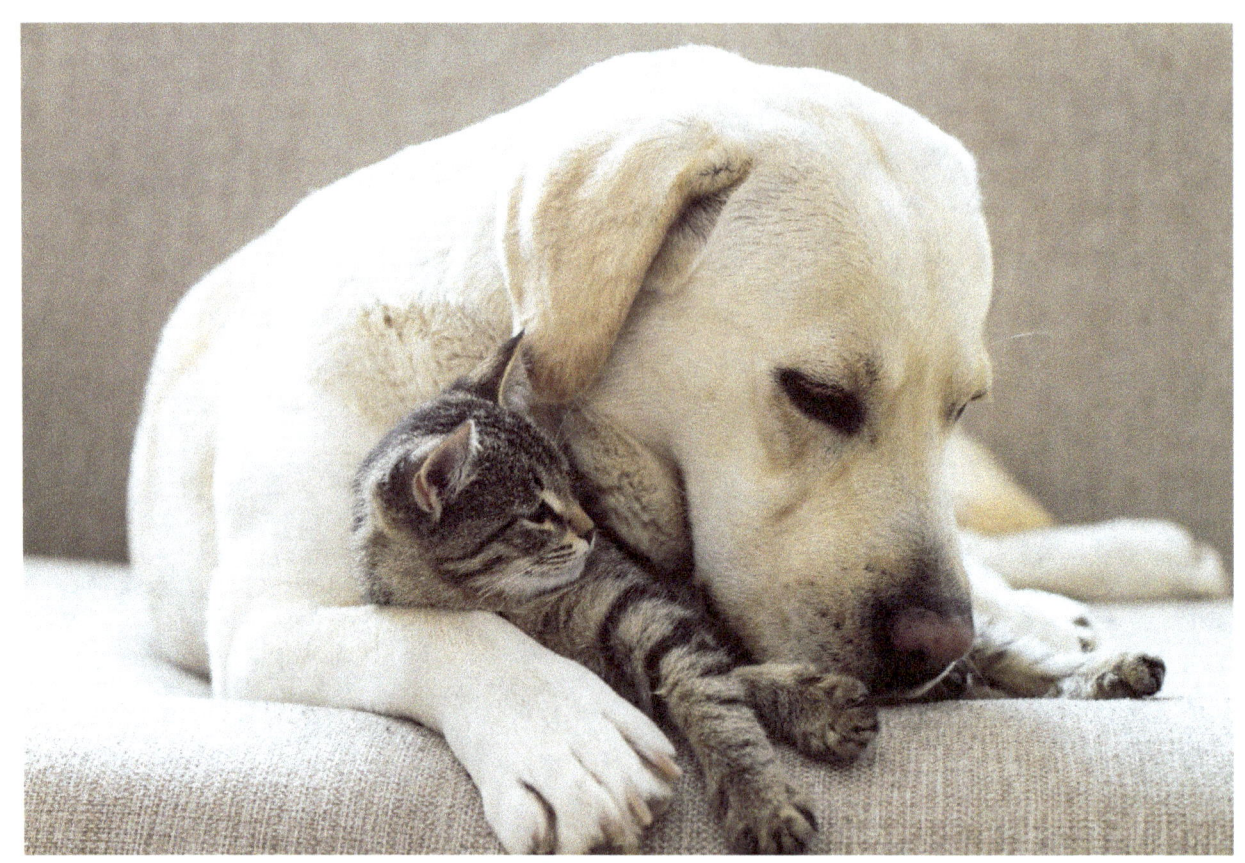

A good friend indeed

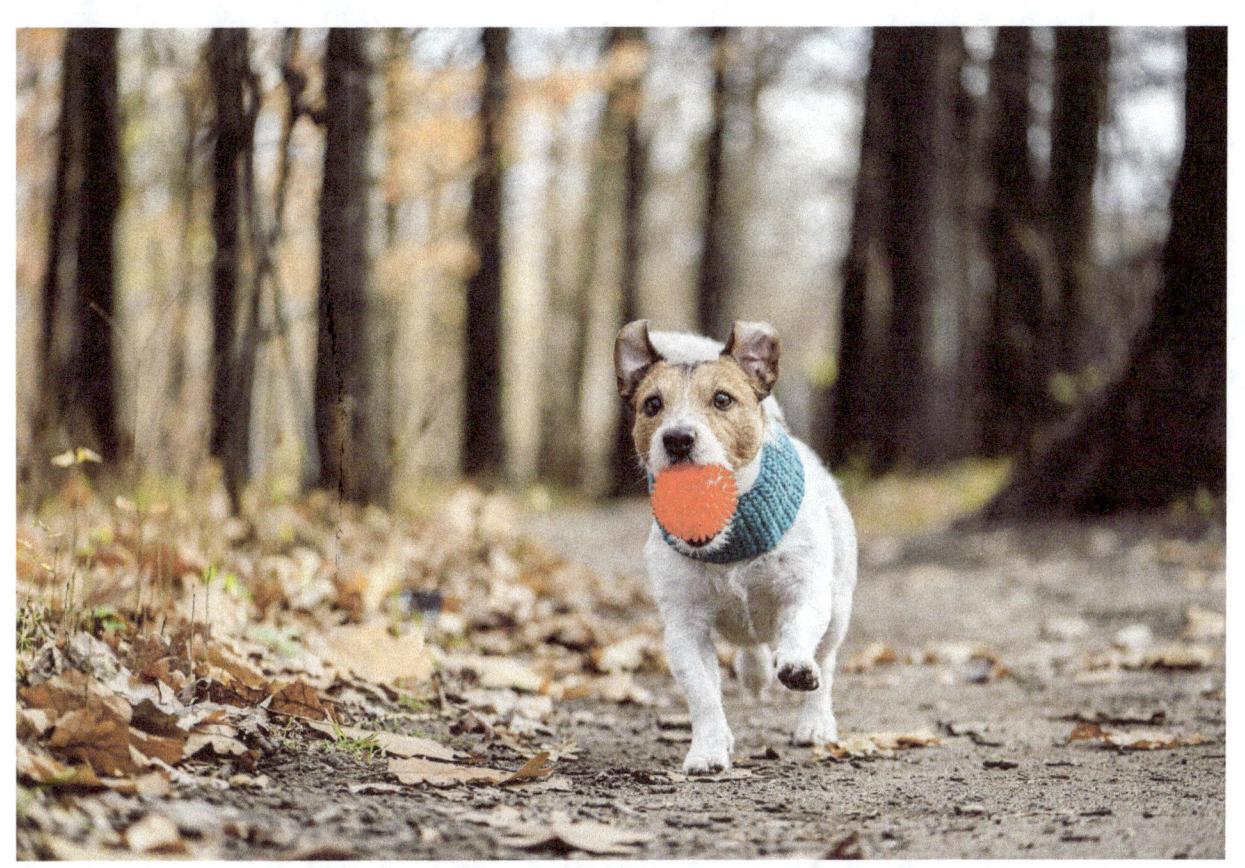

I got the ball!

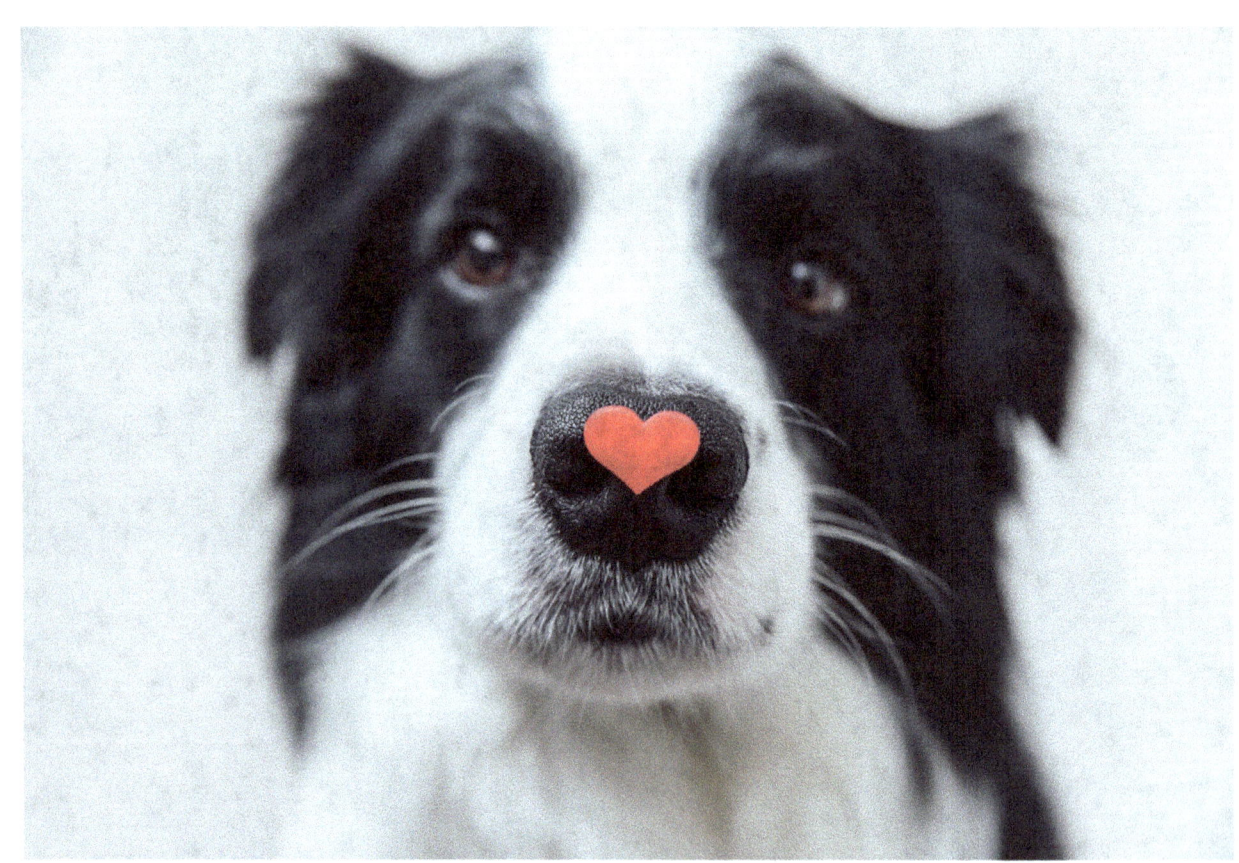

A dog is a man's best friend

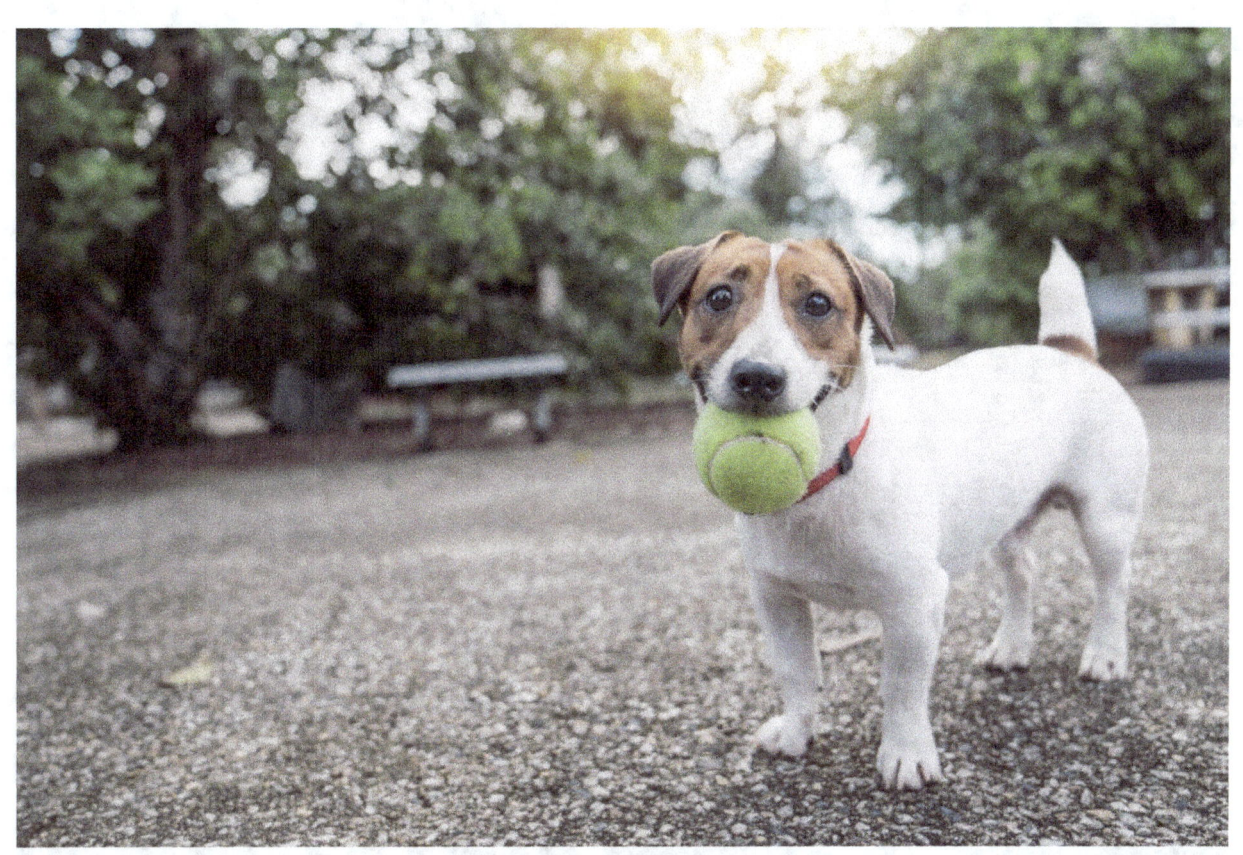

Playing fetch is my favorite!

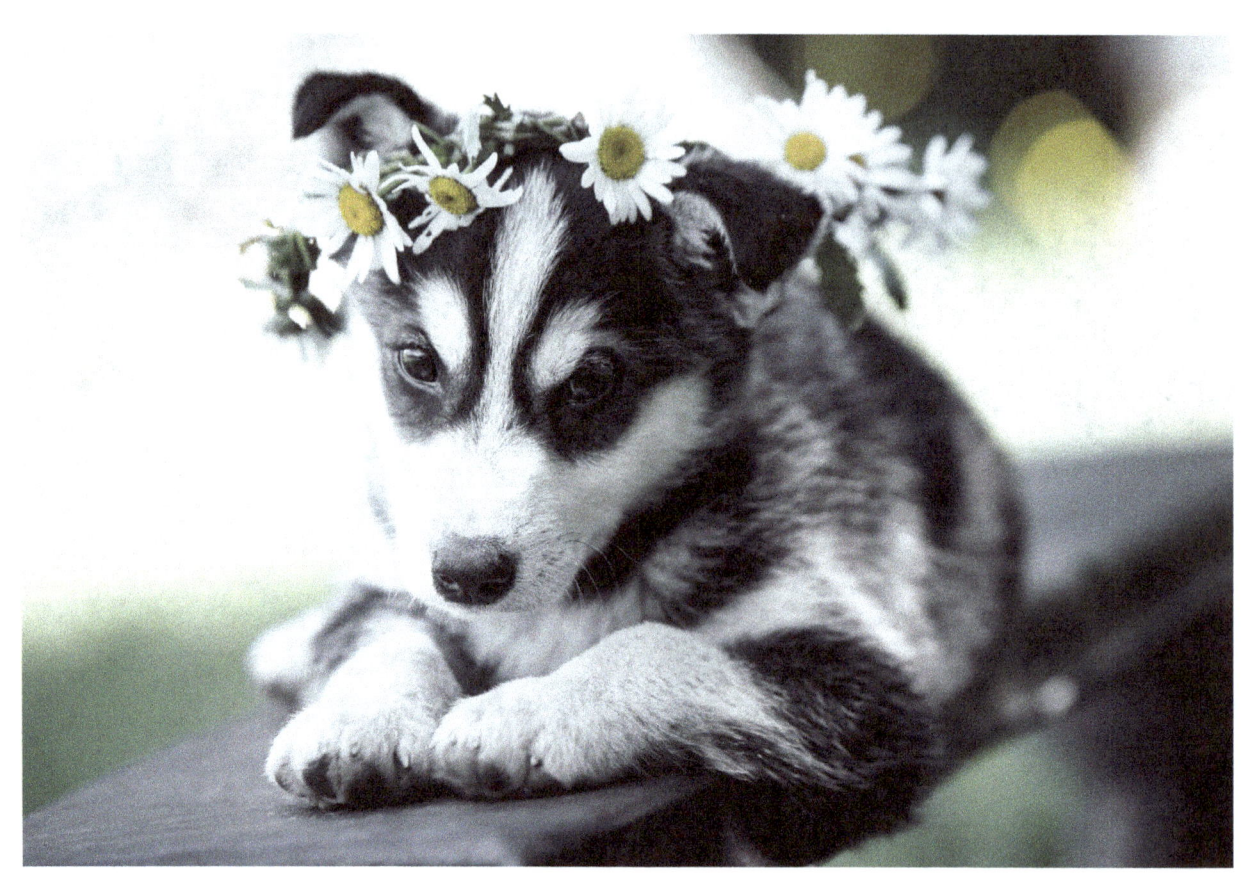

A crown of daisies

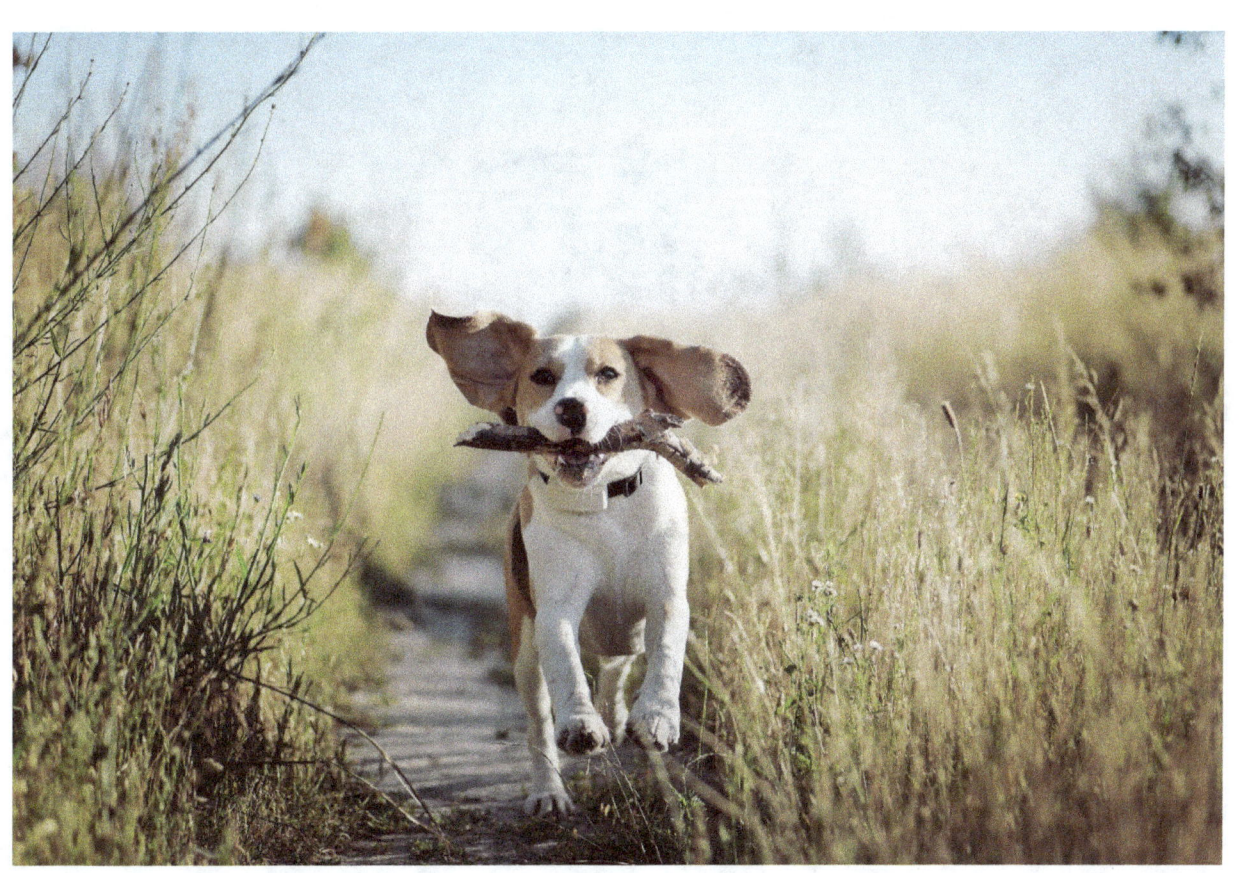

Summer sun on the run!

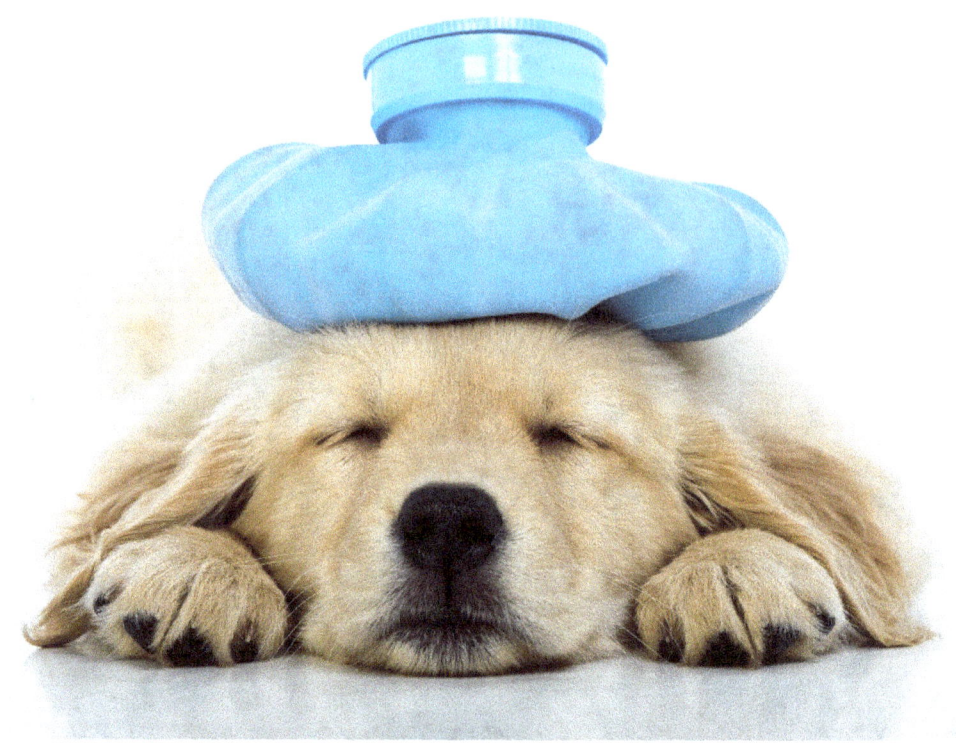

Aaaaaah.

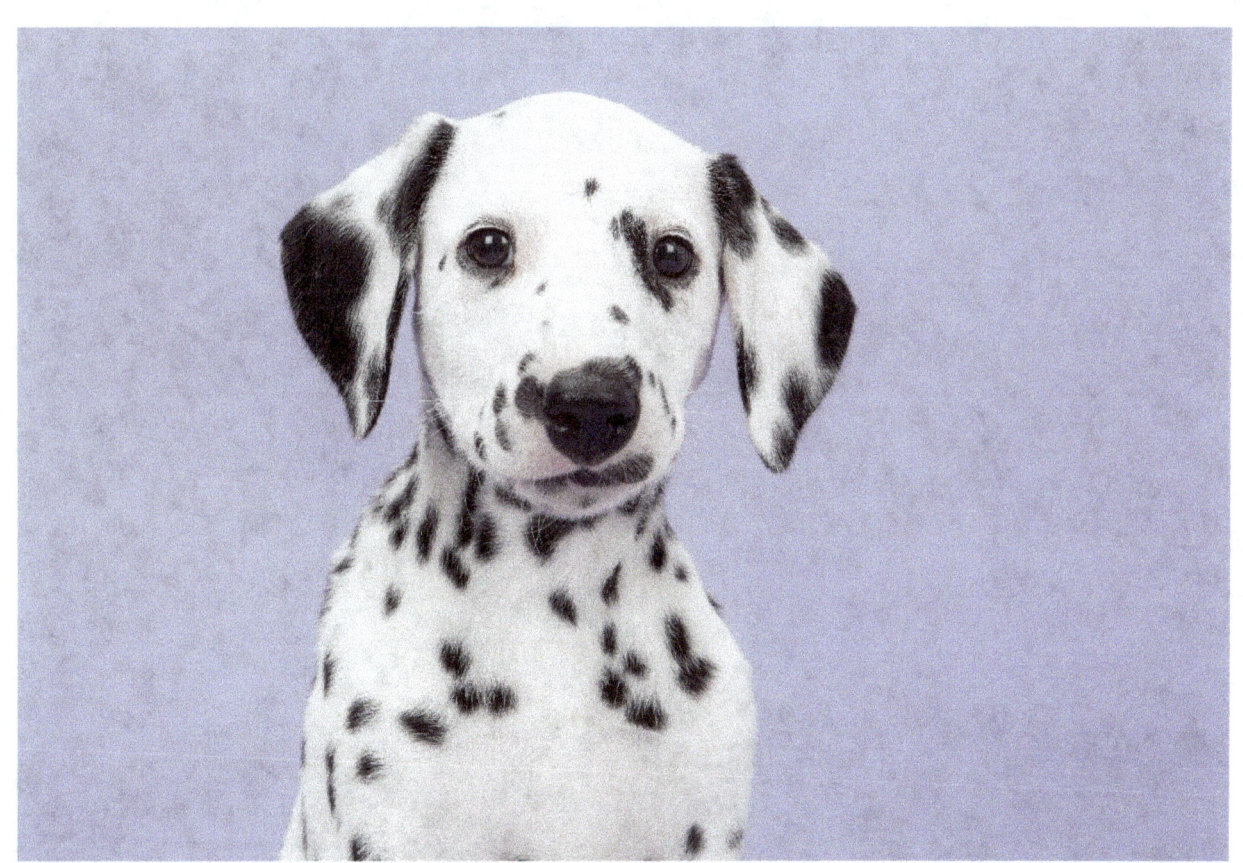

Polka dots

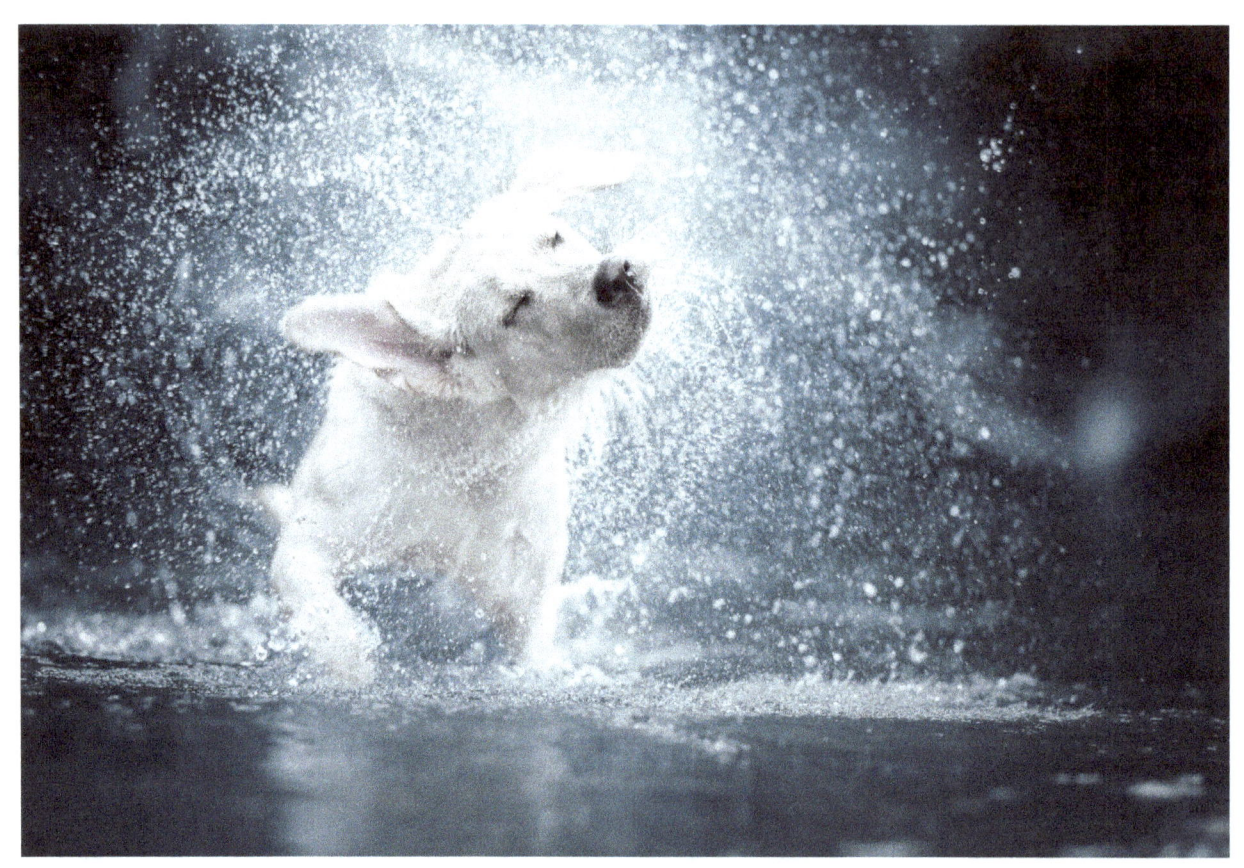

A good swim!

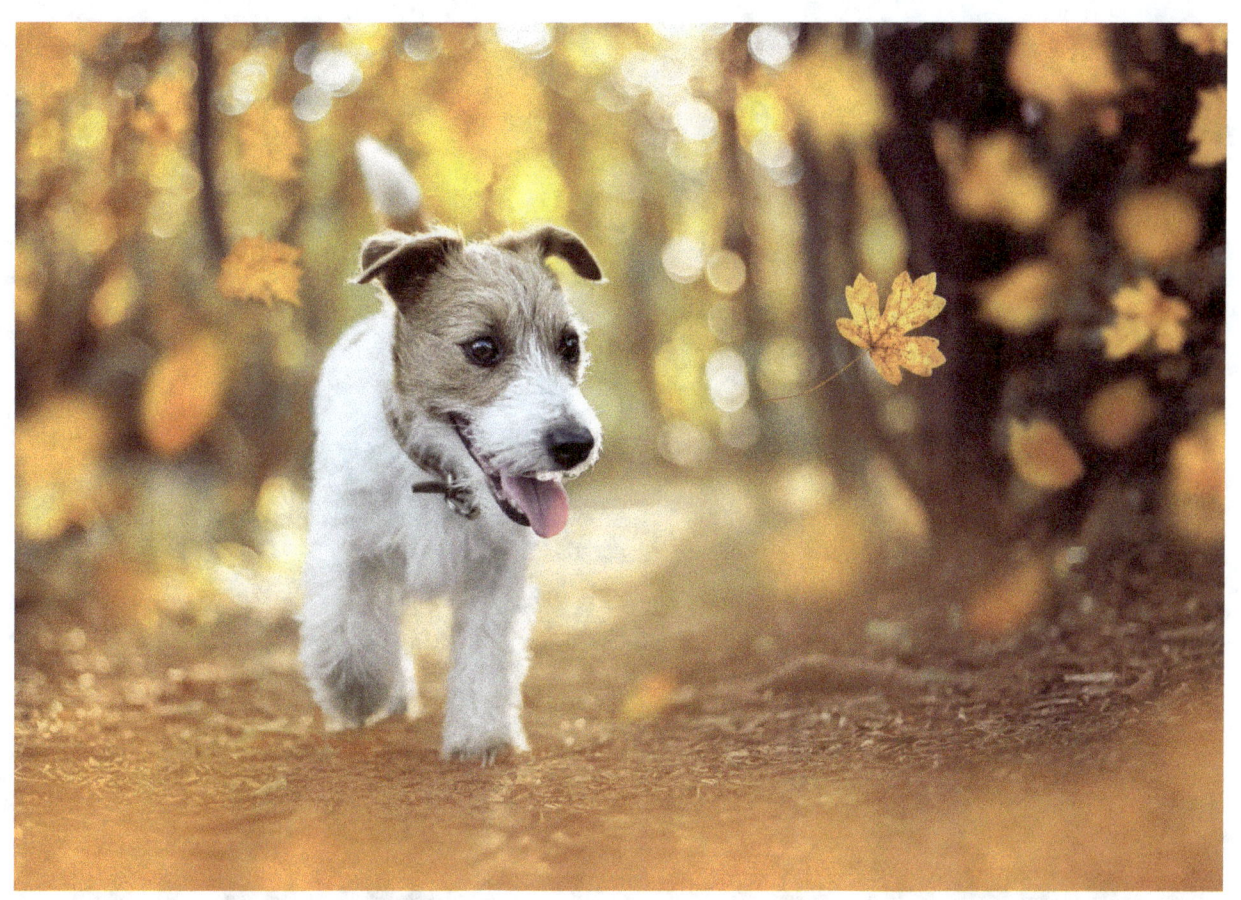

Autumn trails a blazing

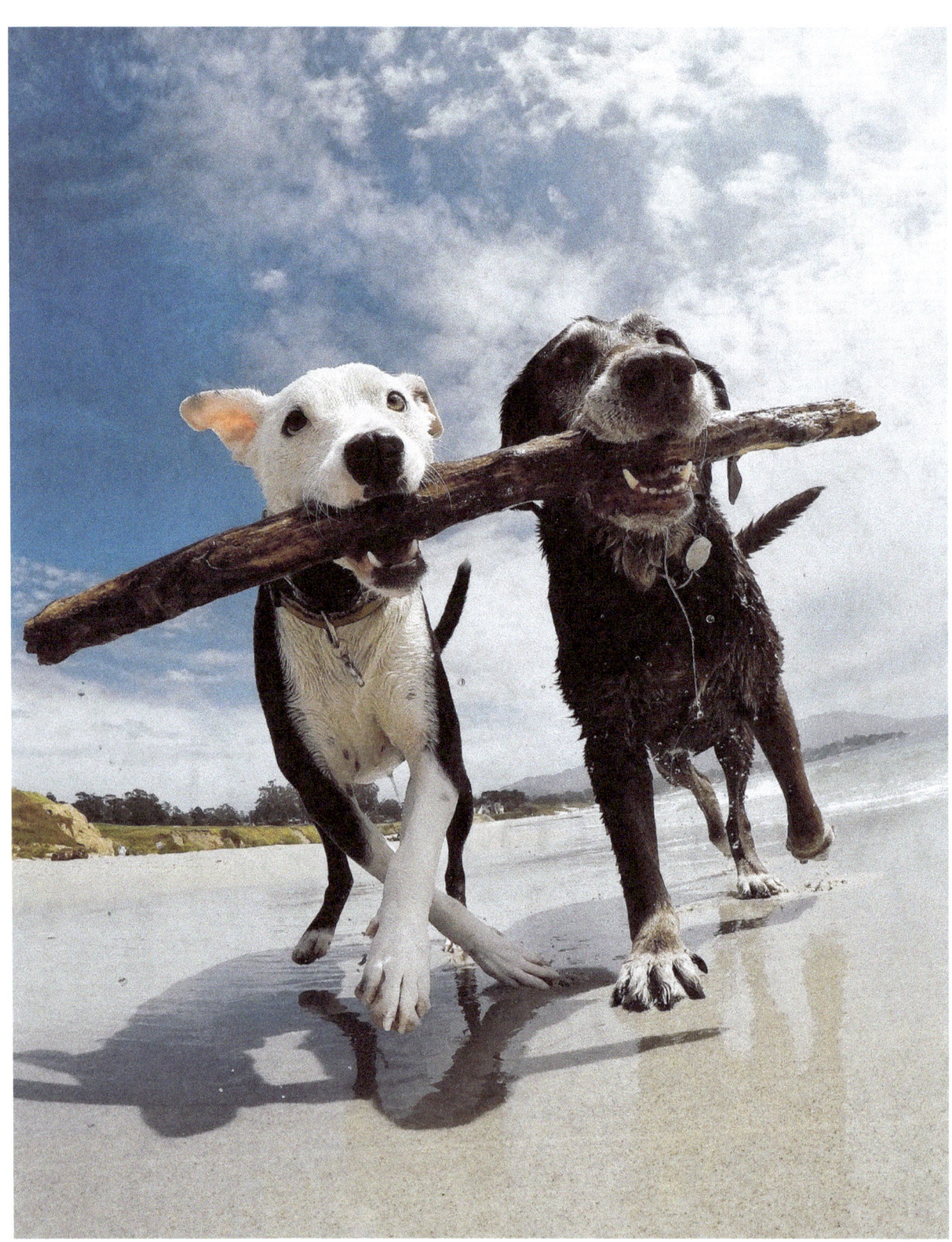

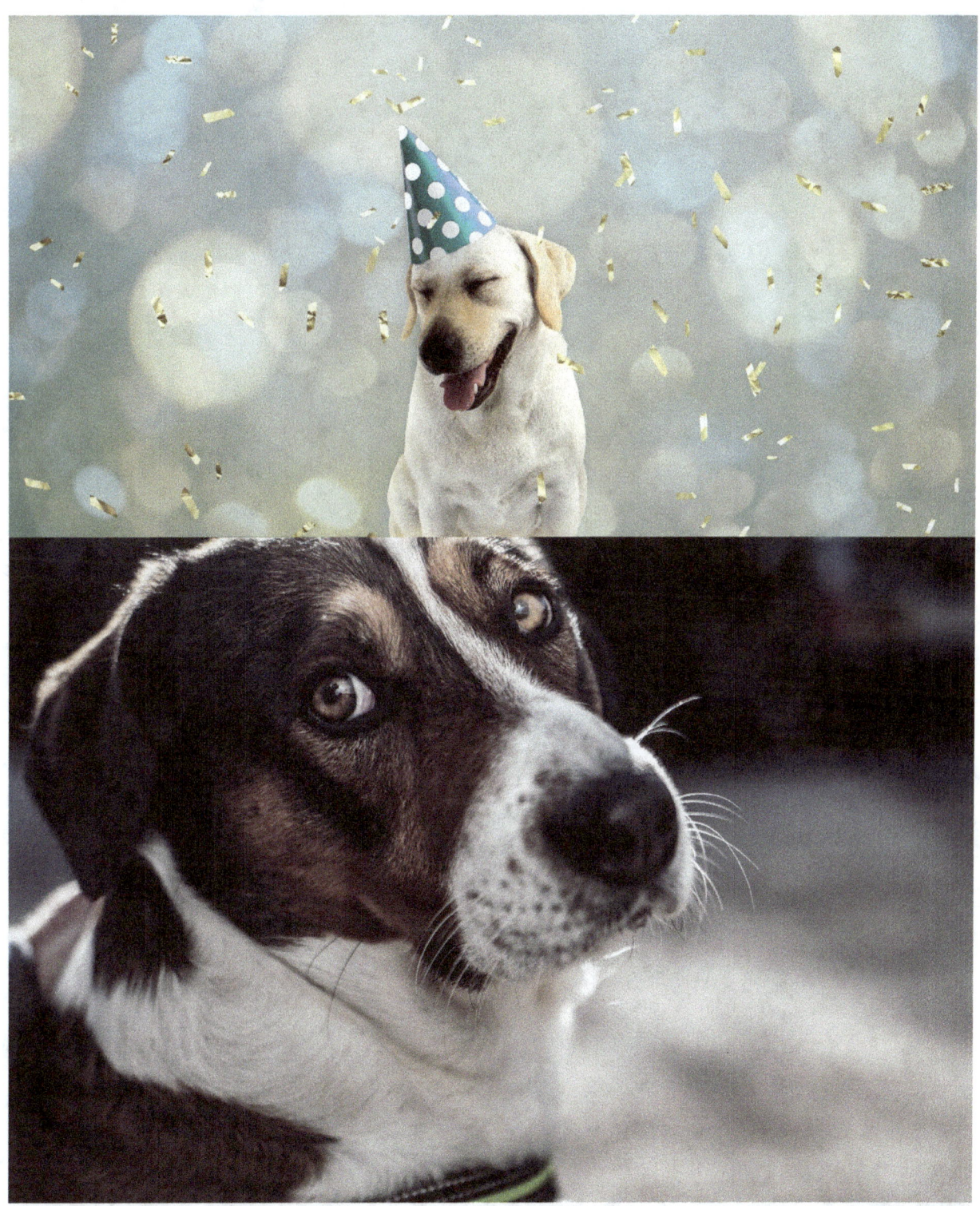

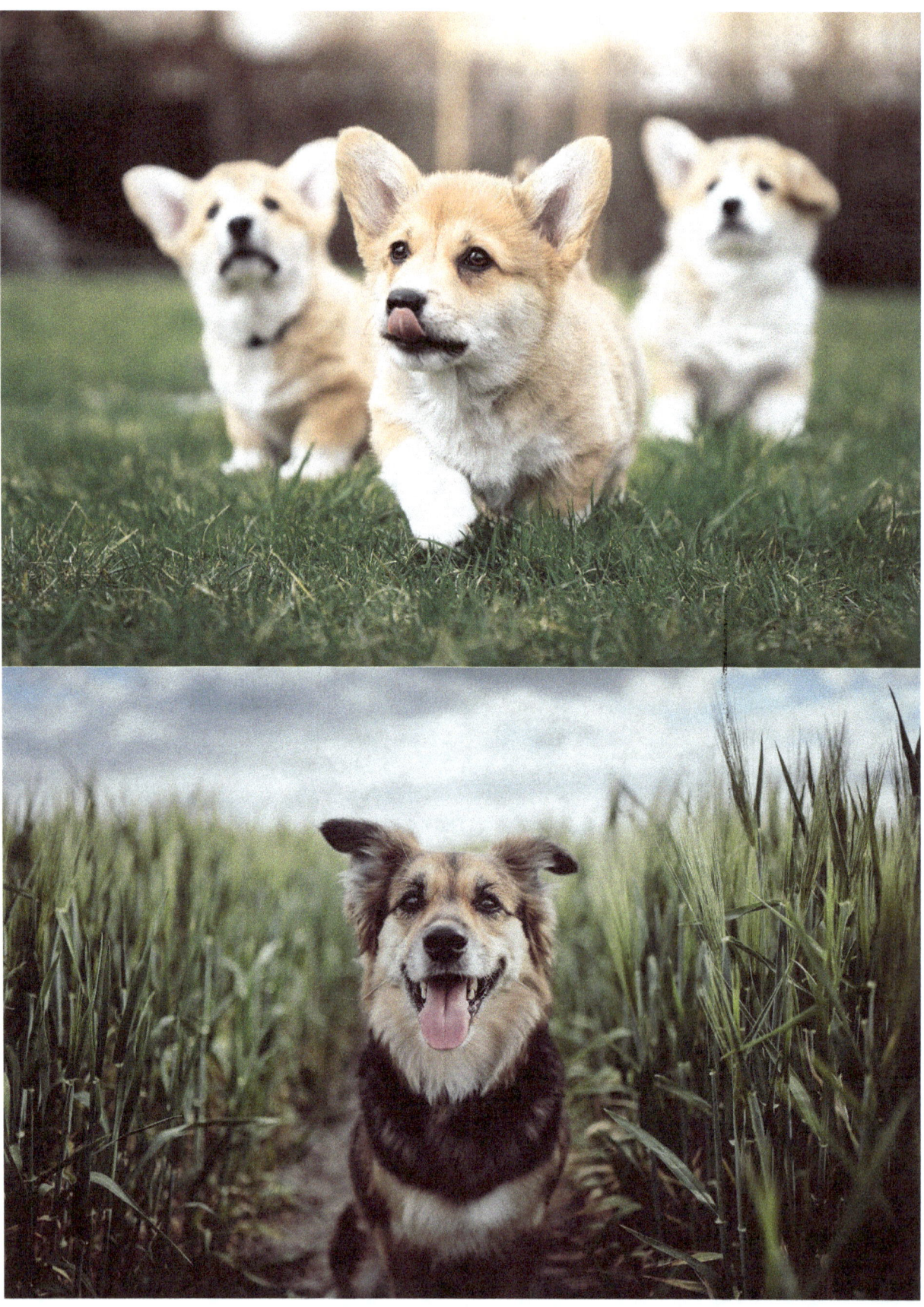

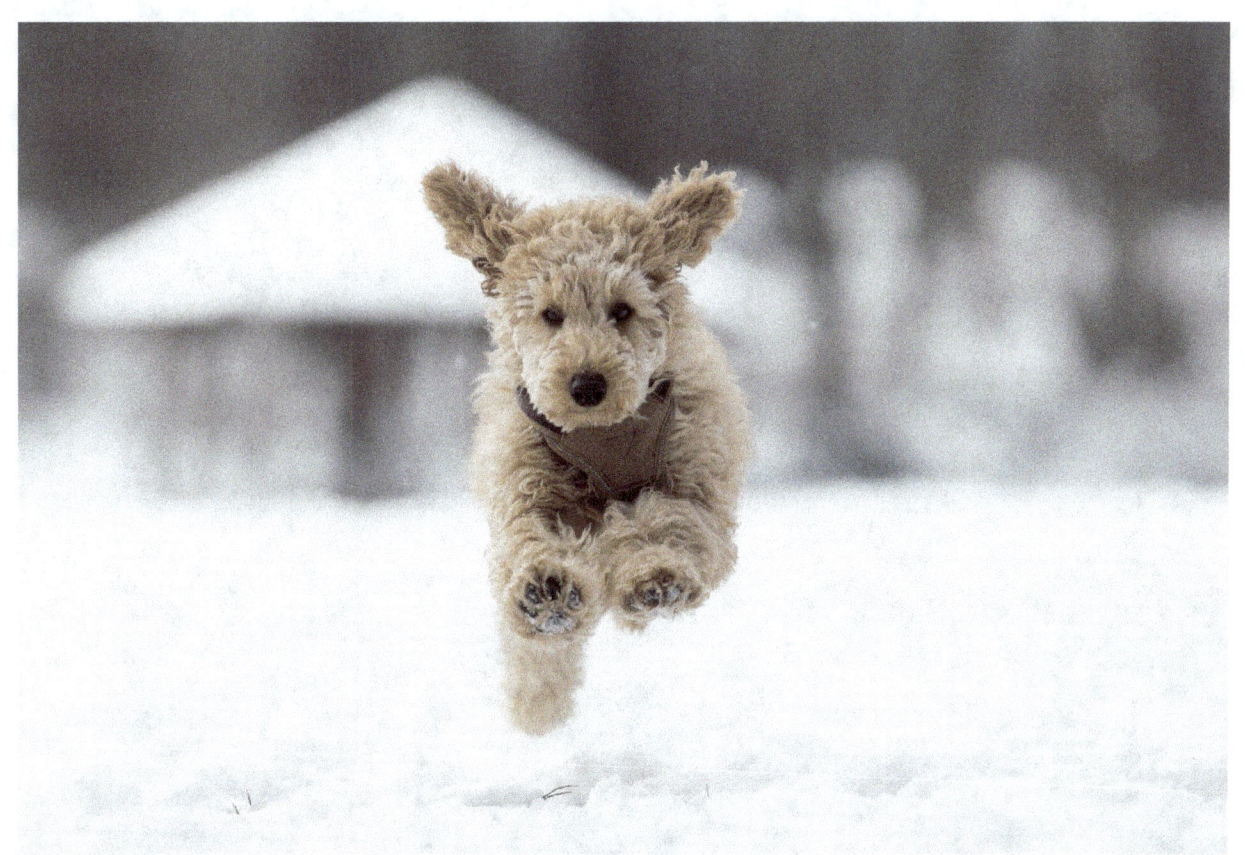

Weeeeeeeeeee!

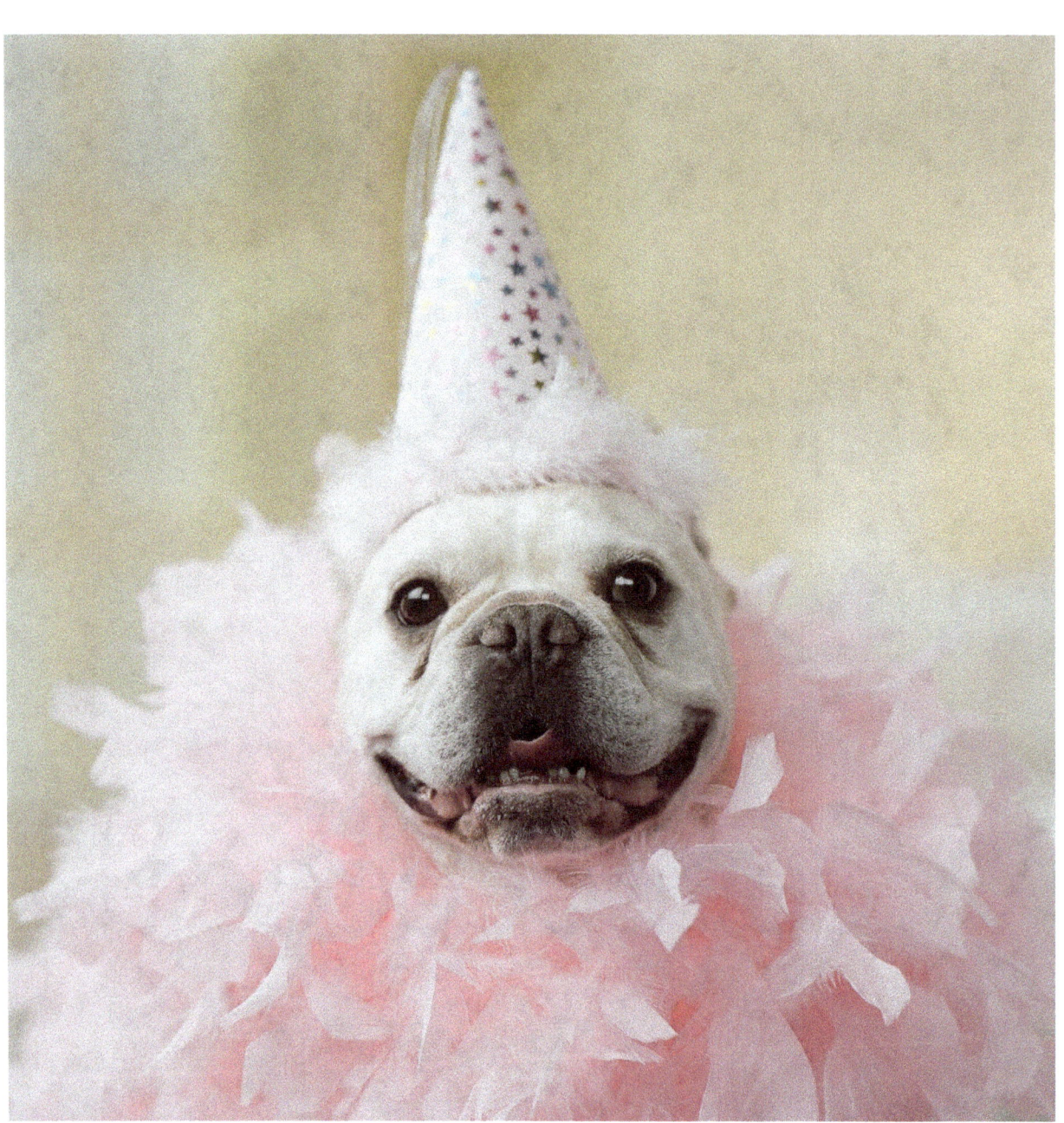

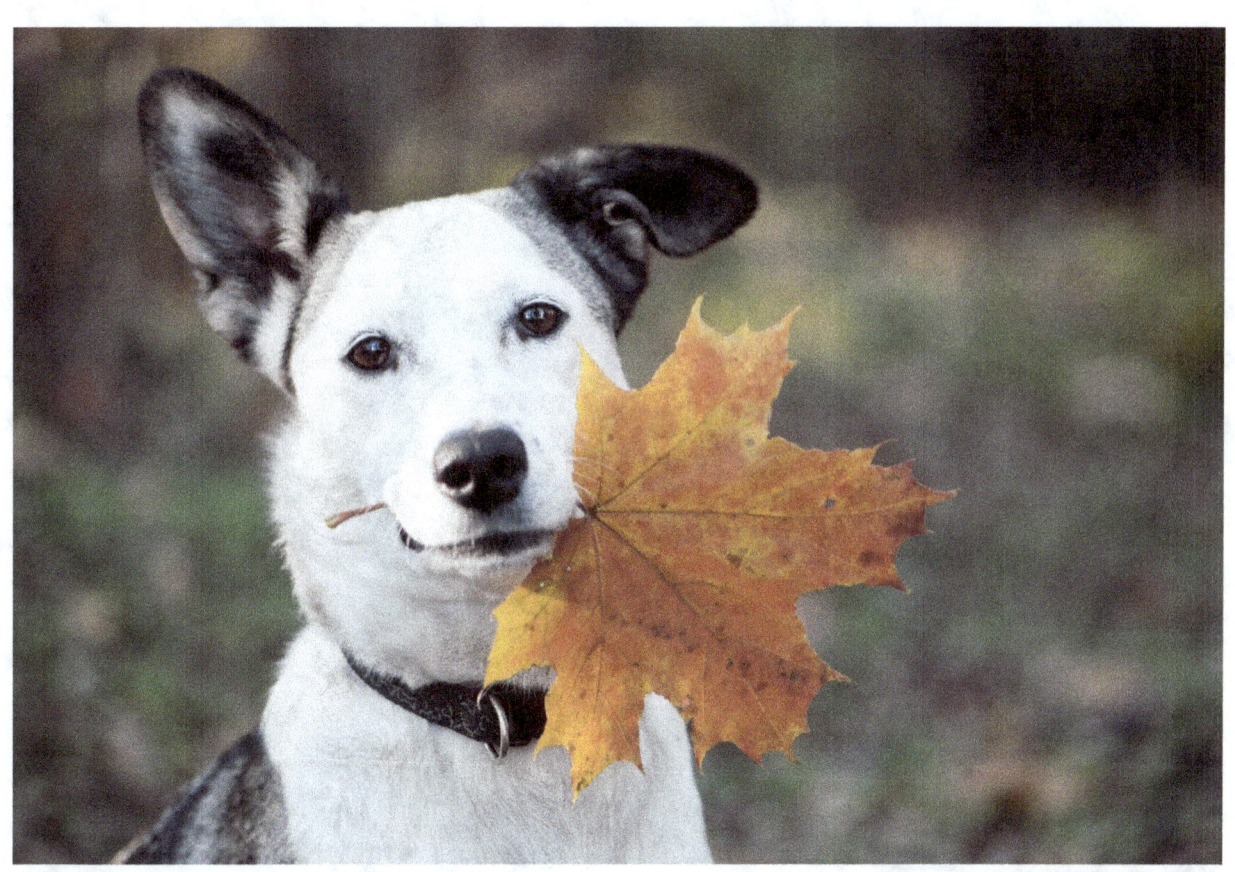

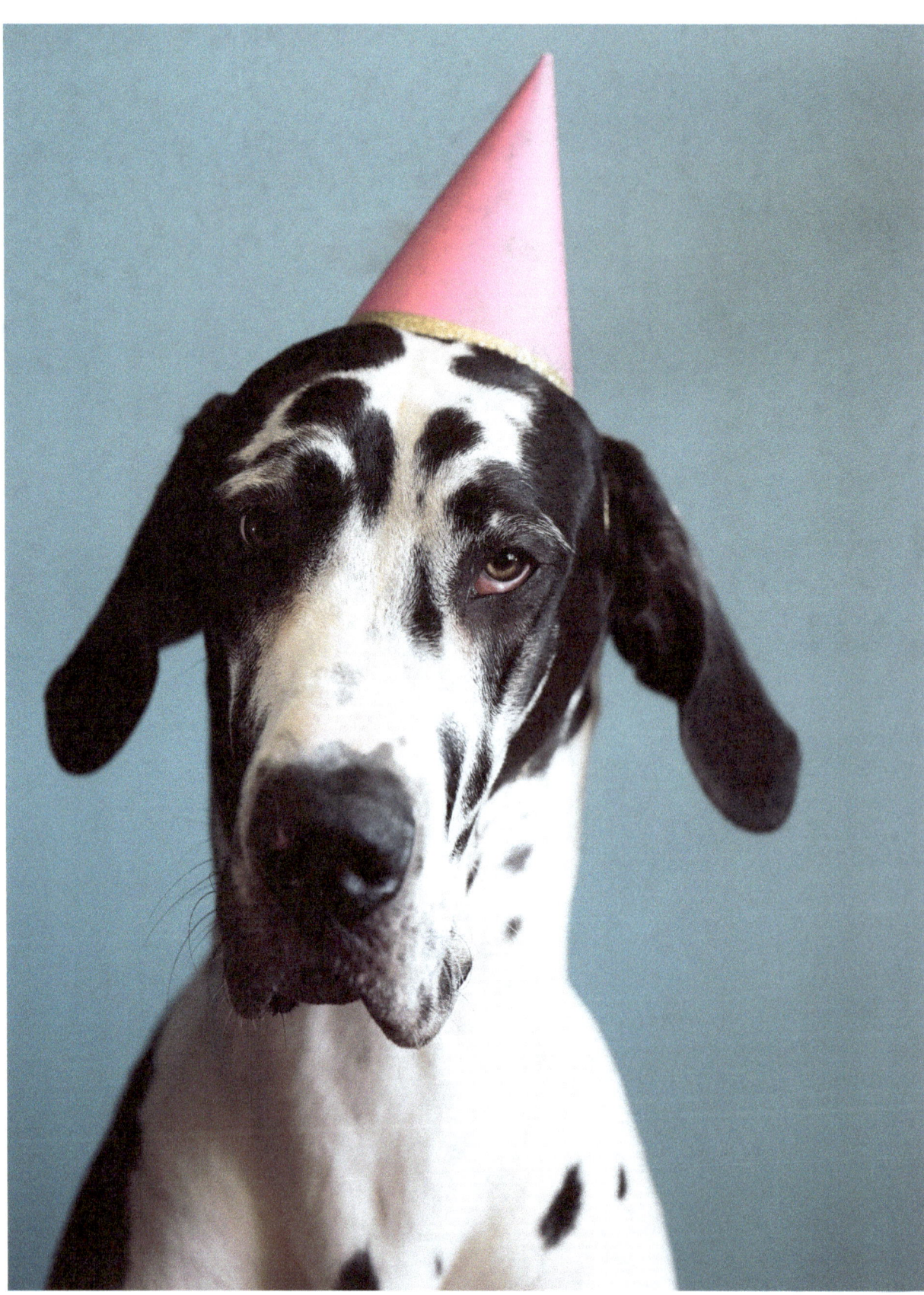

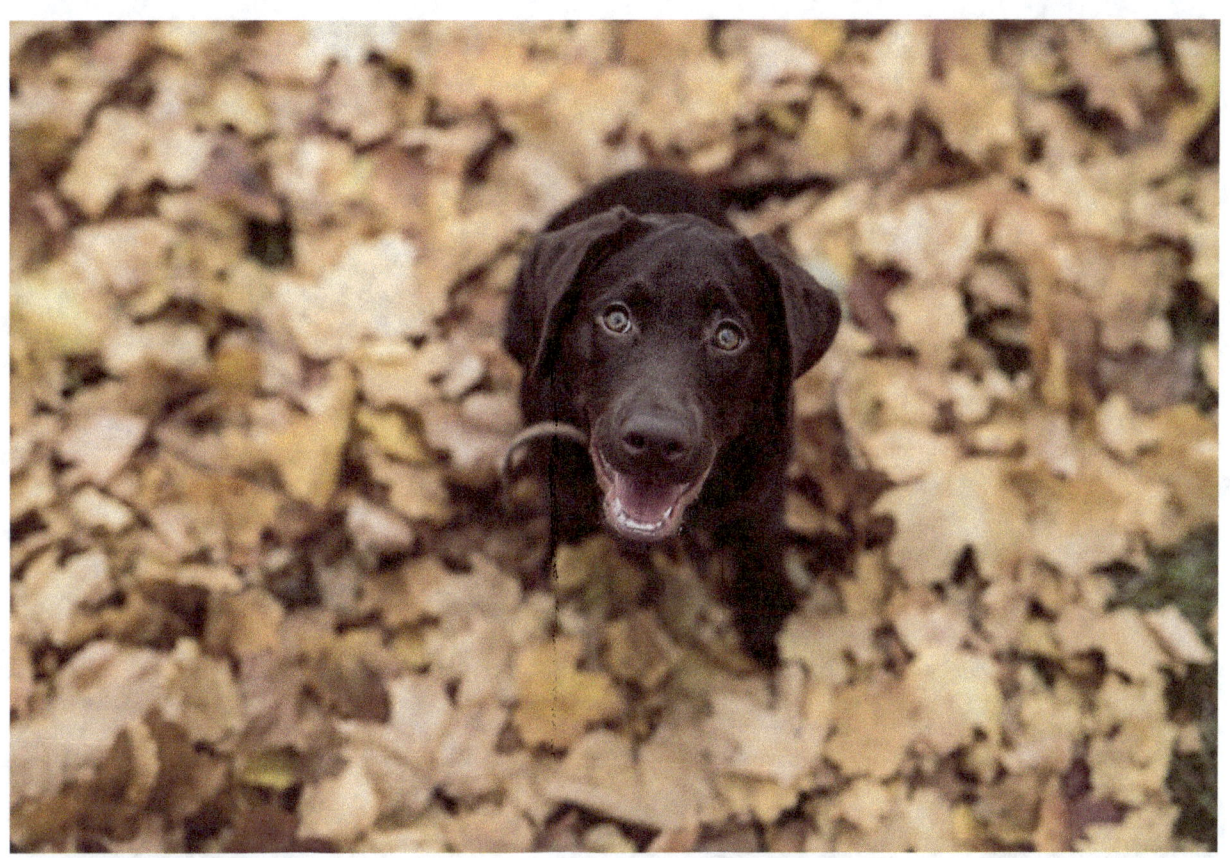

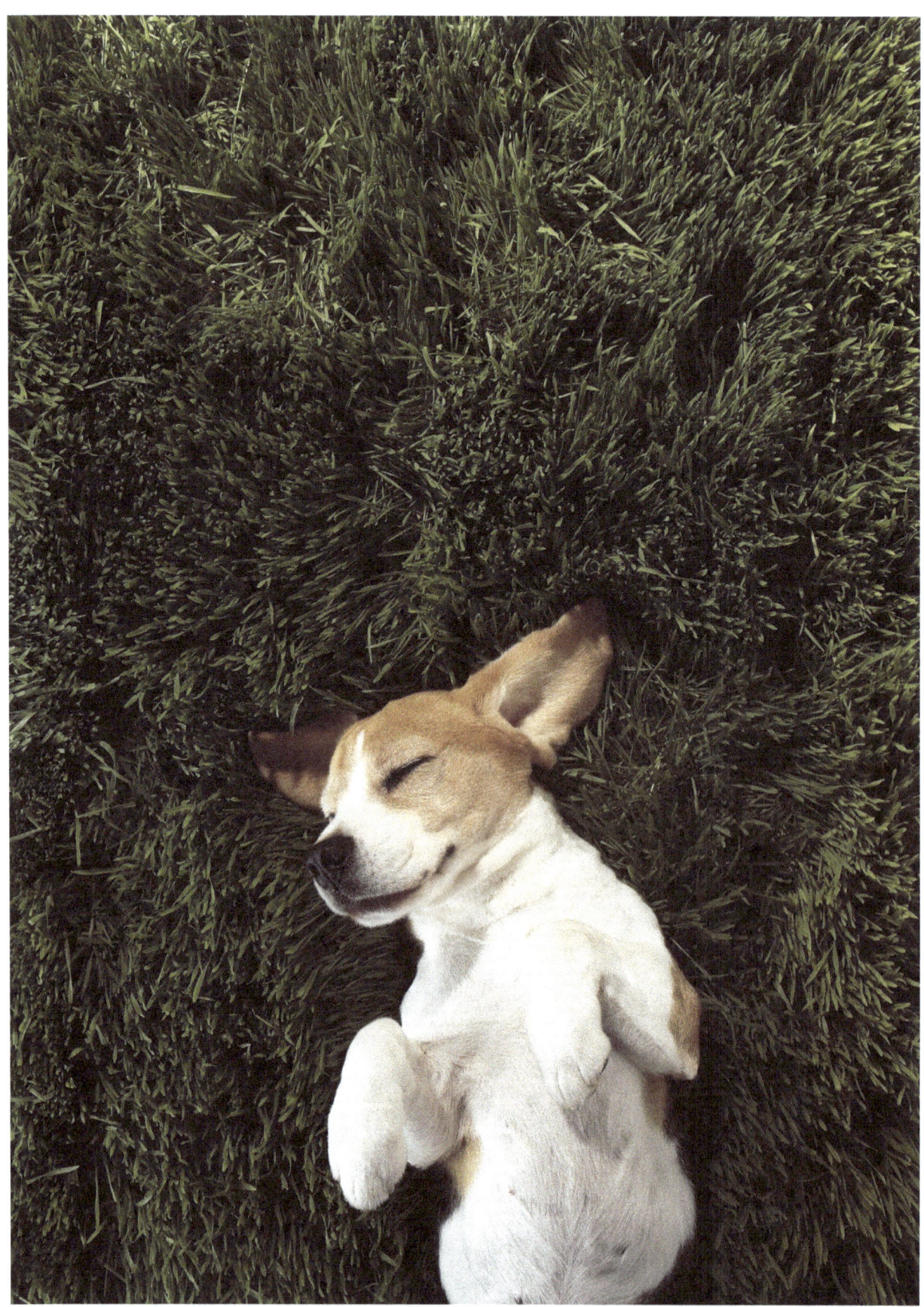

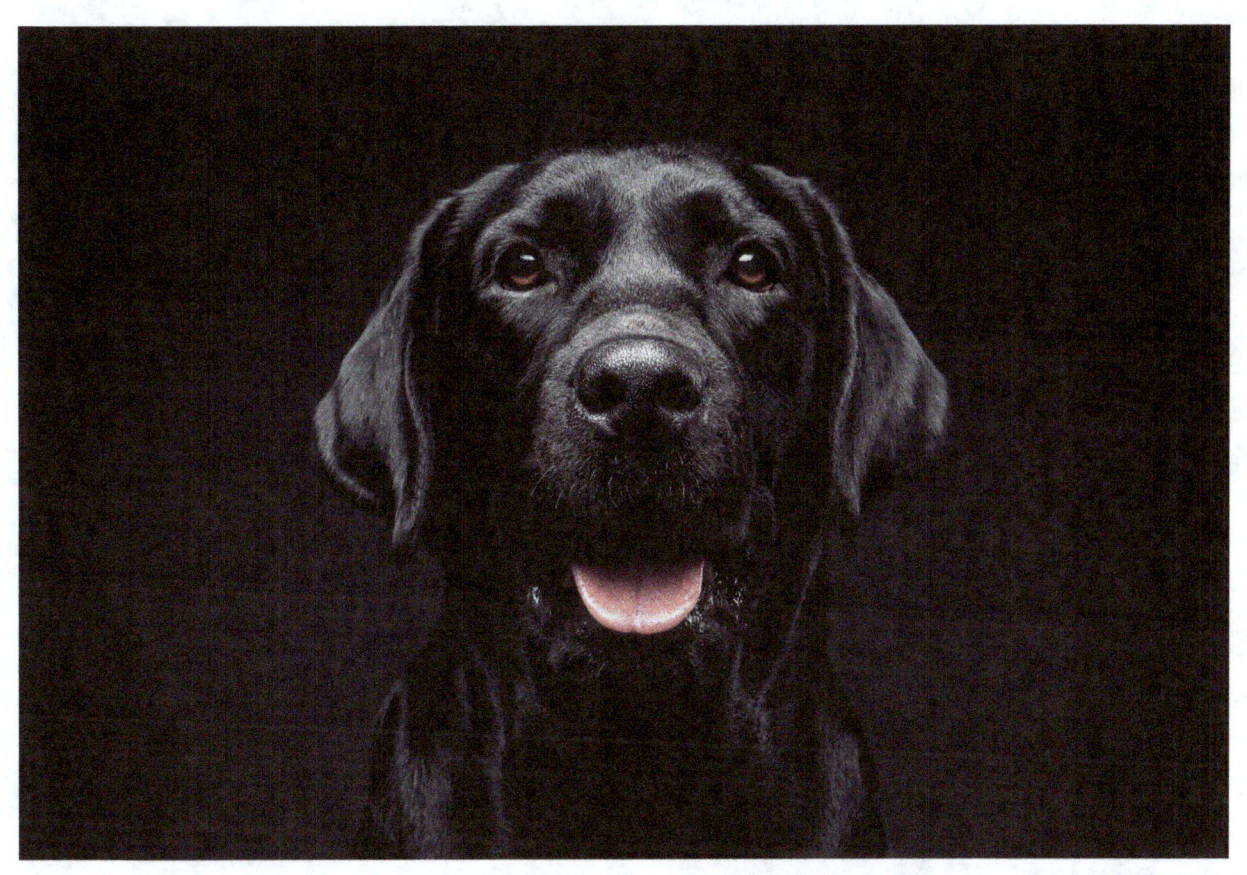

I am a very
good boy.

Water:

Rolling rivers ~

Serene lakes ~

Gushing

waterfalls

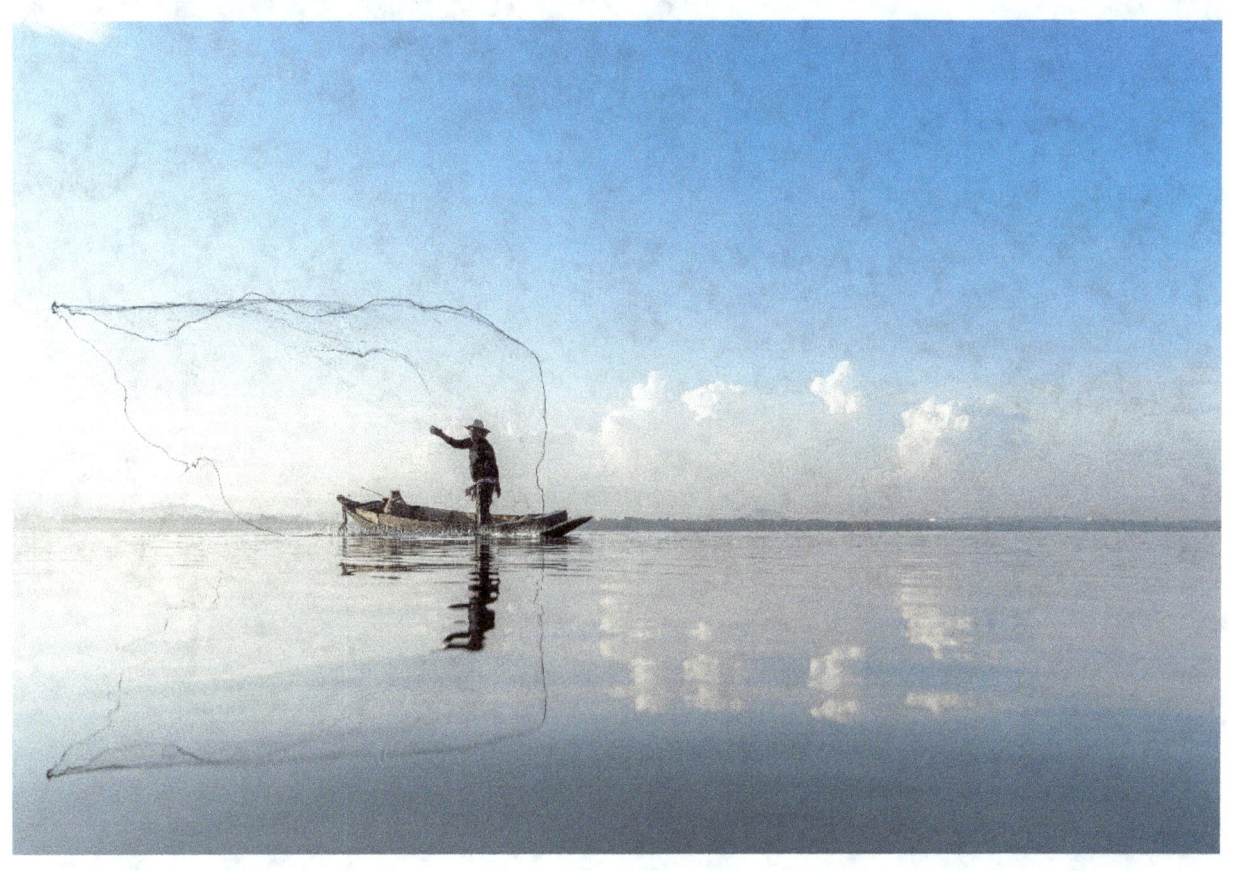

Let's go fishing

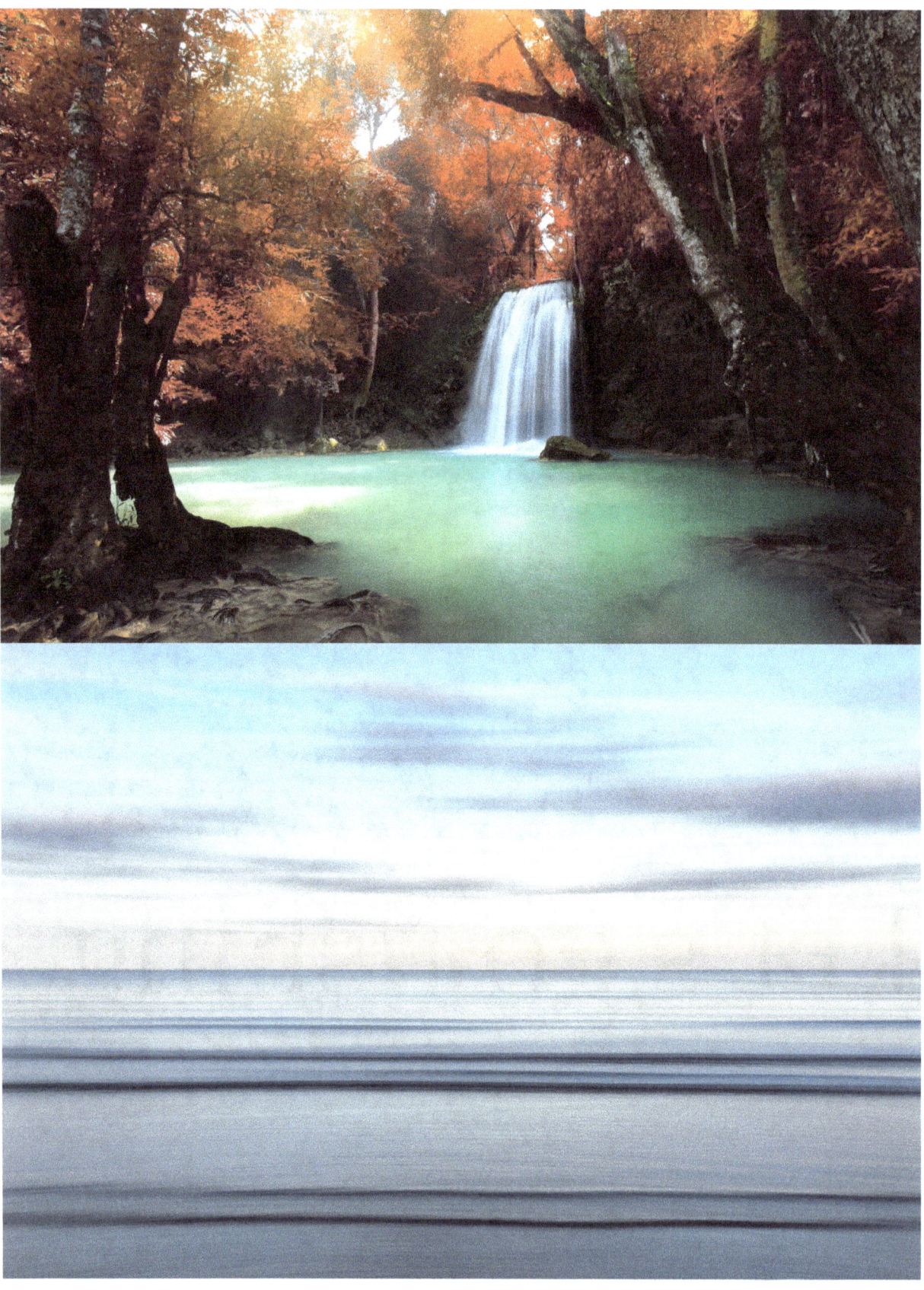

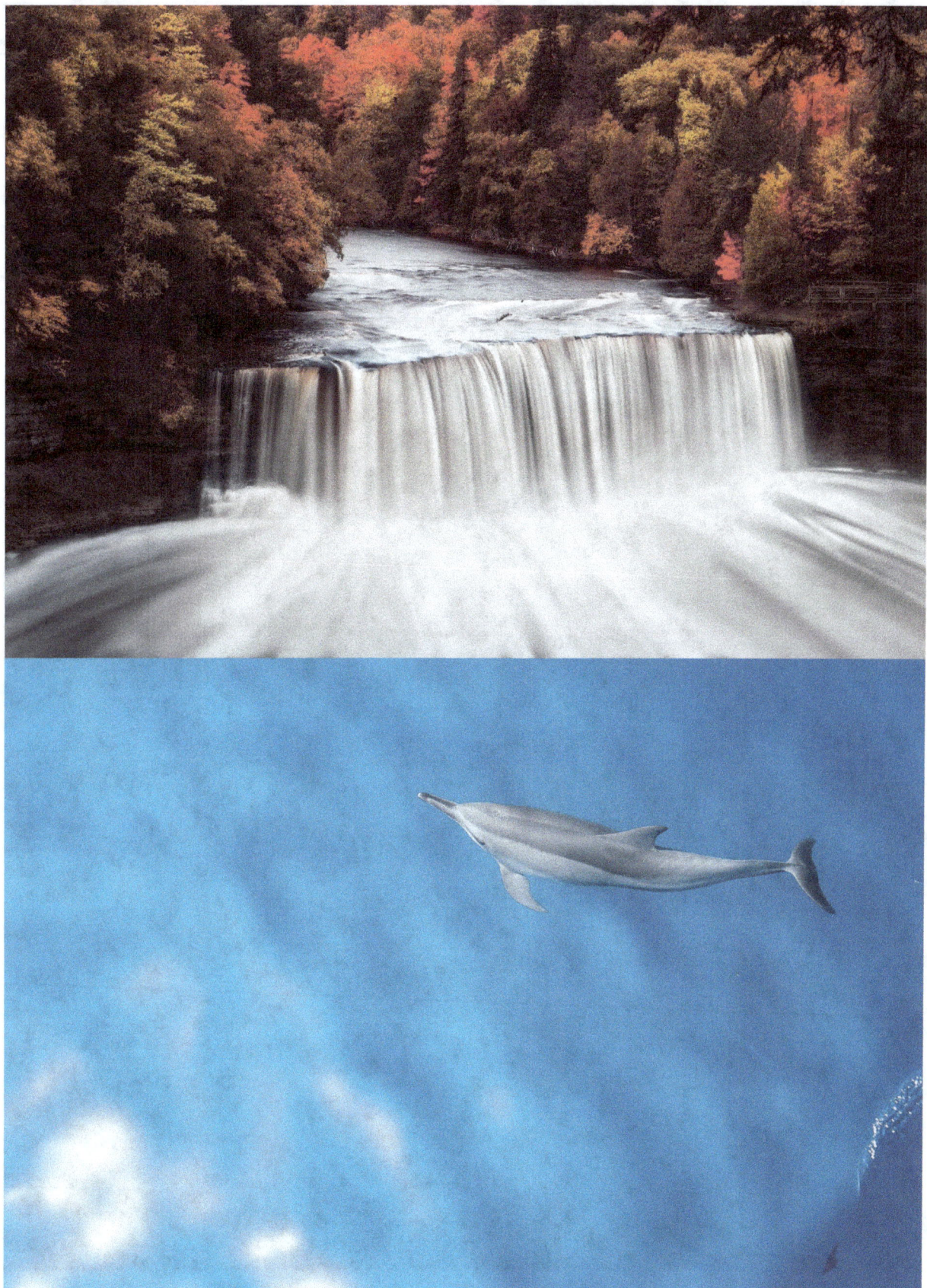

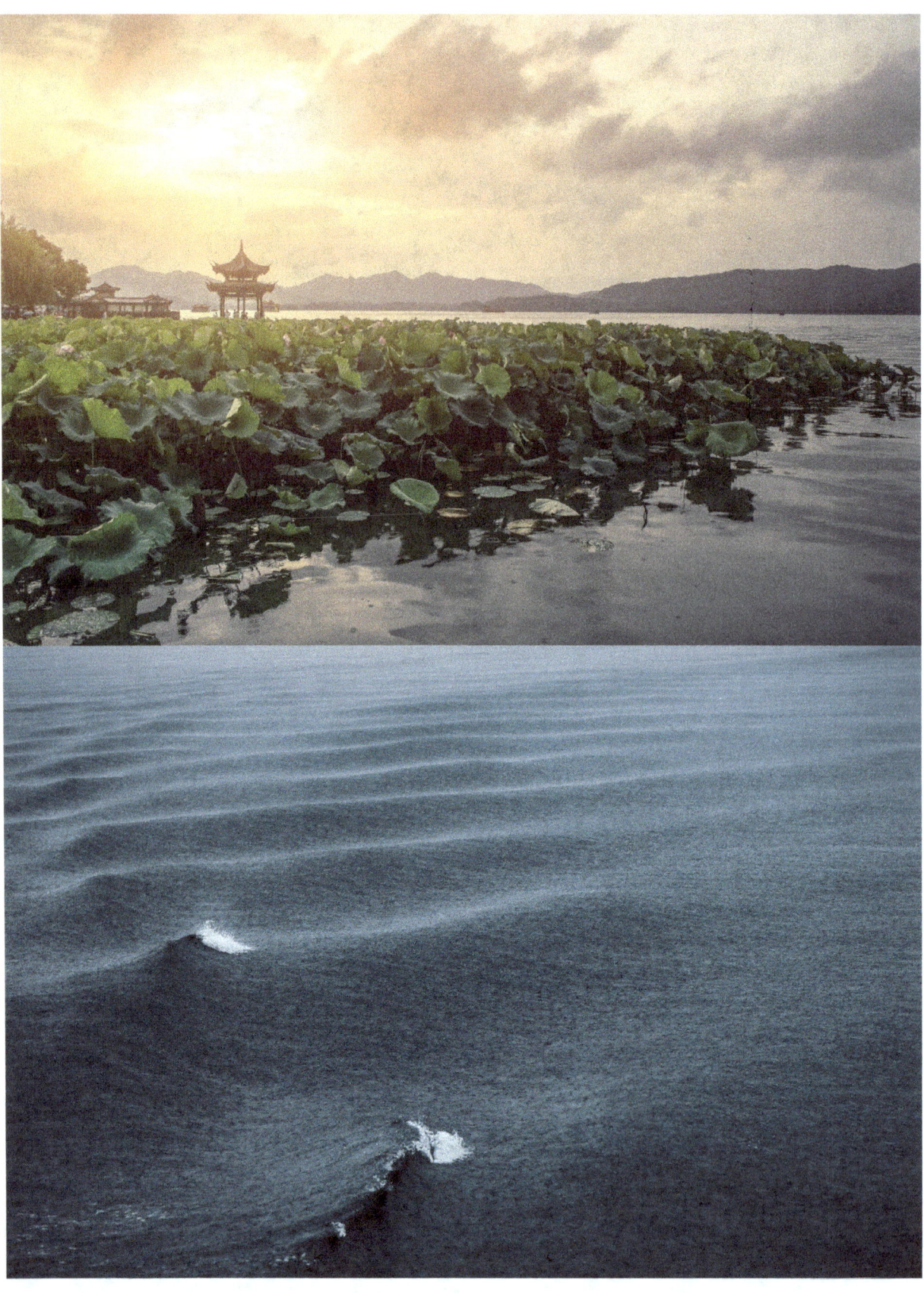

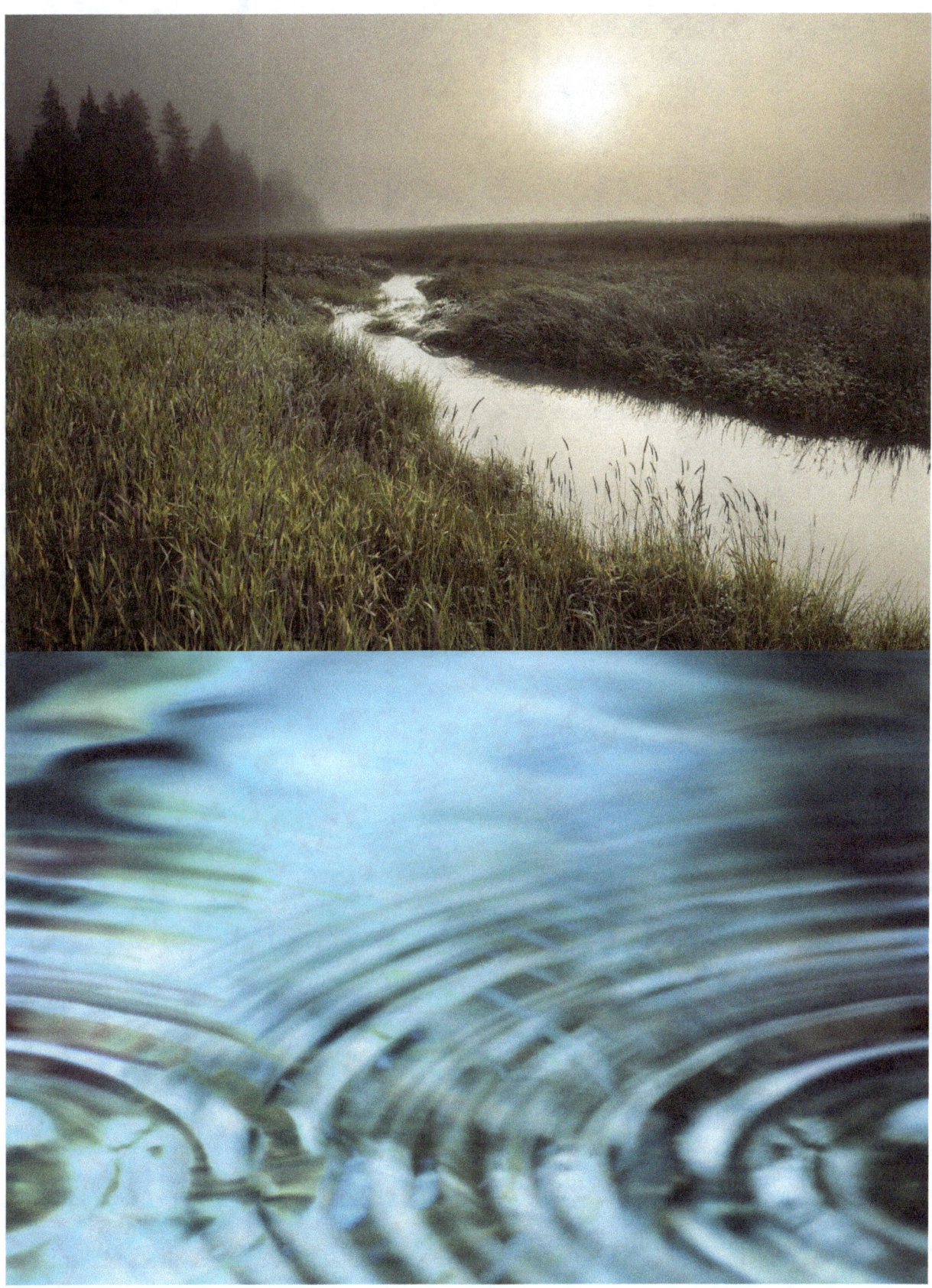

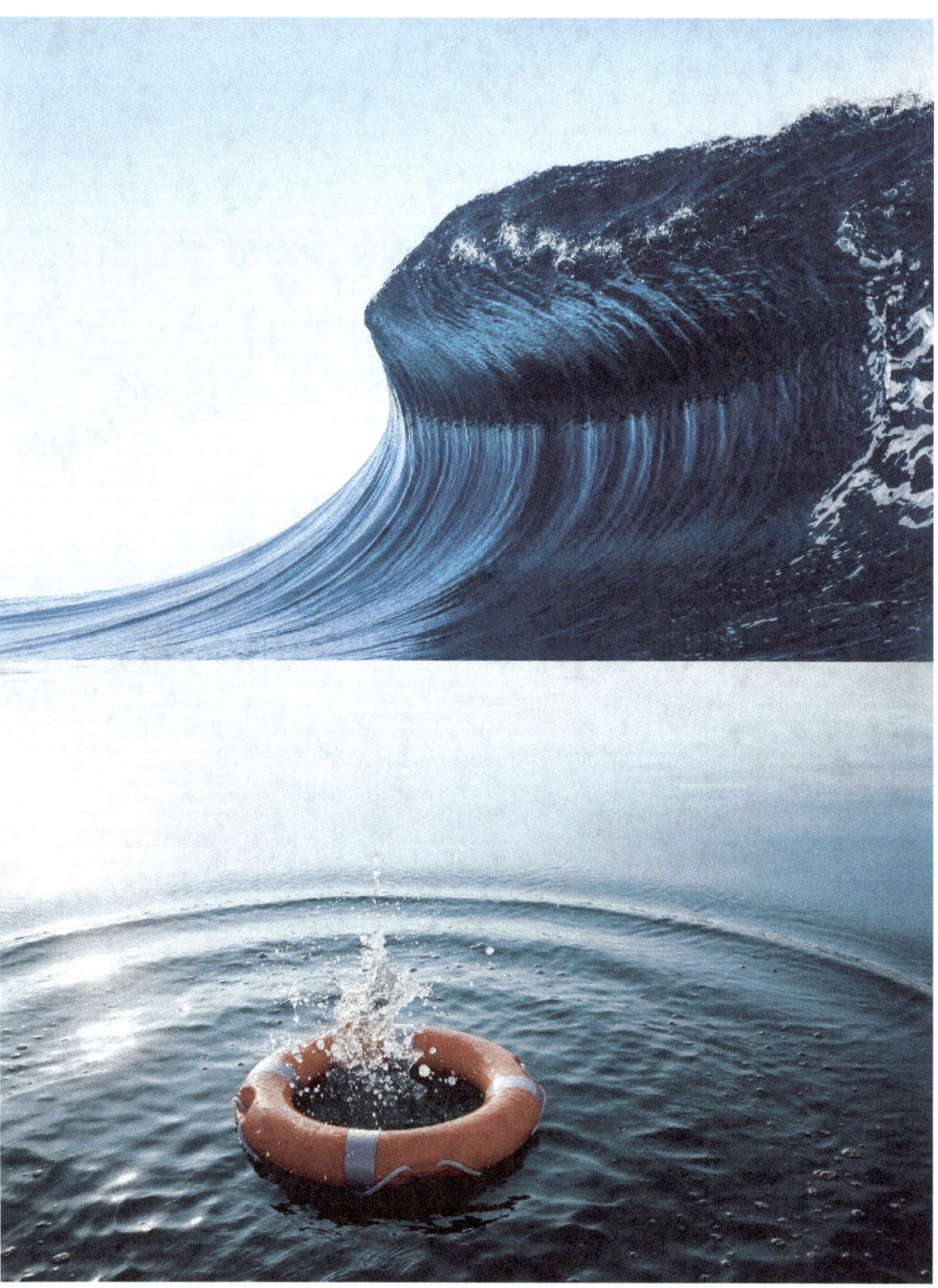

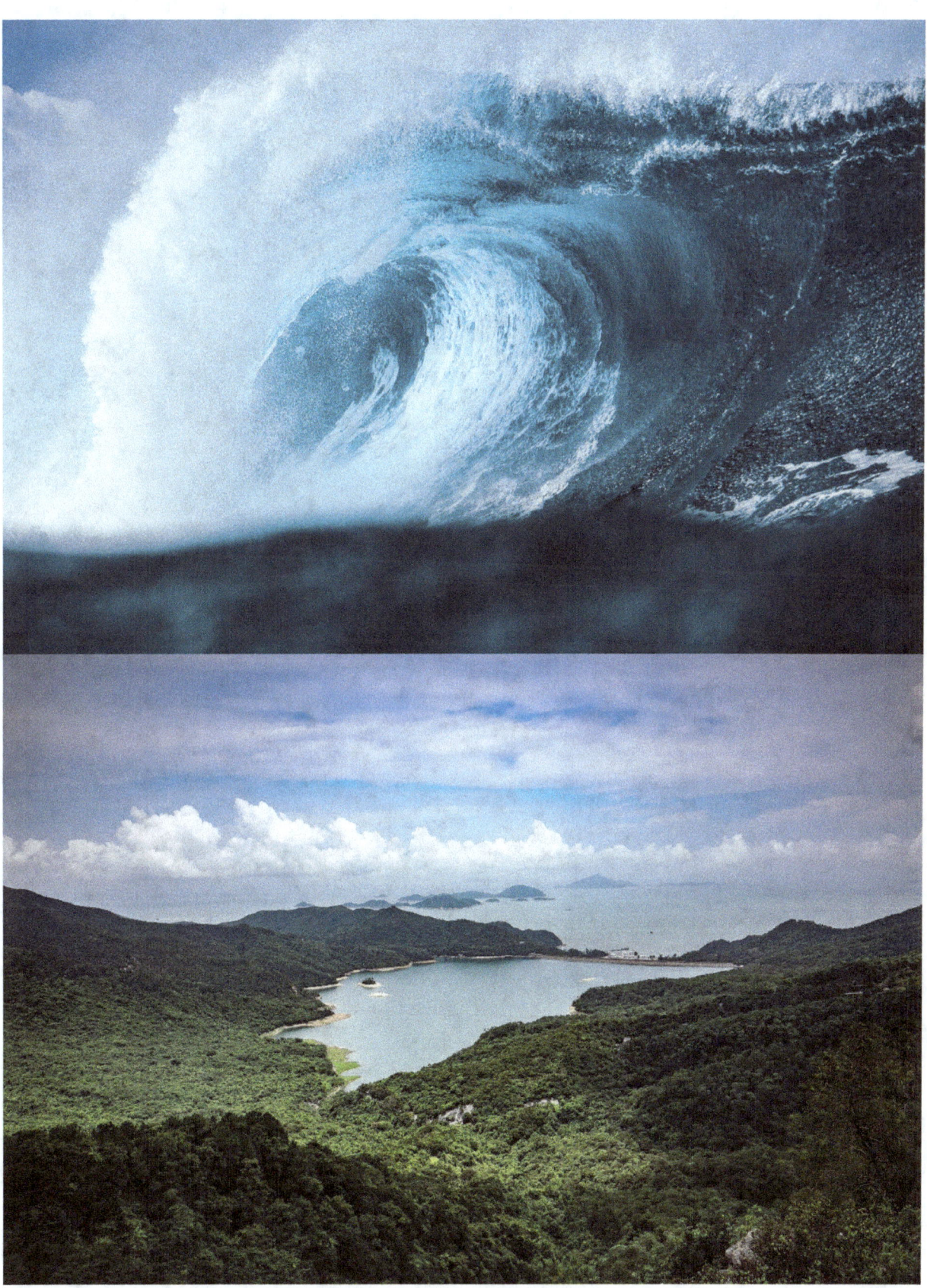

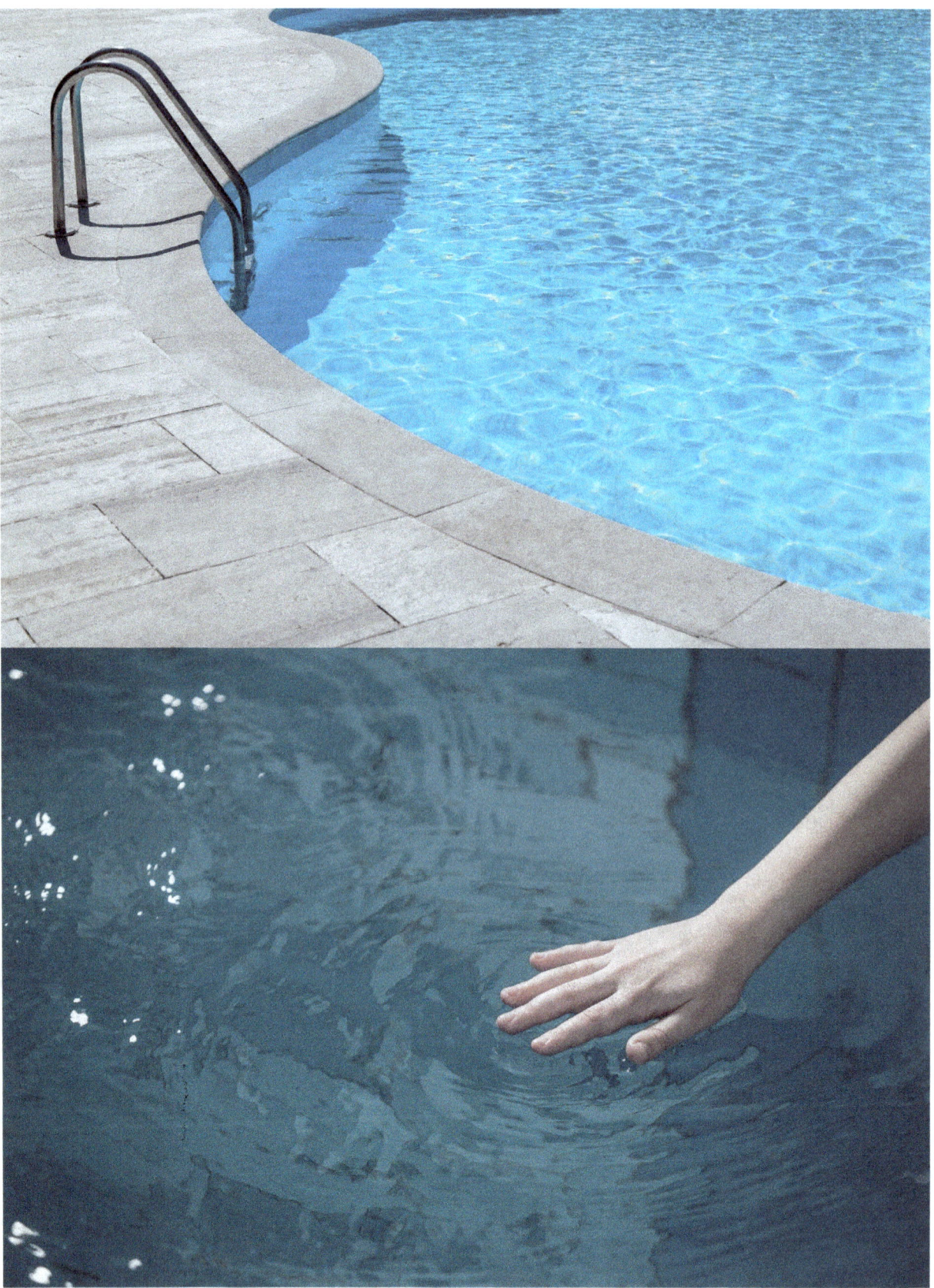

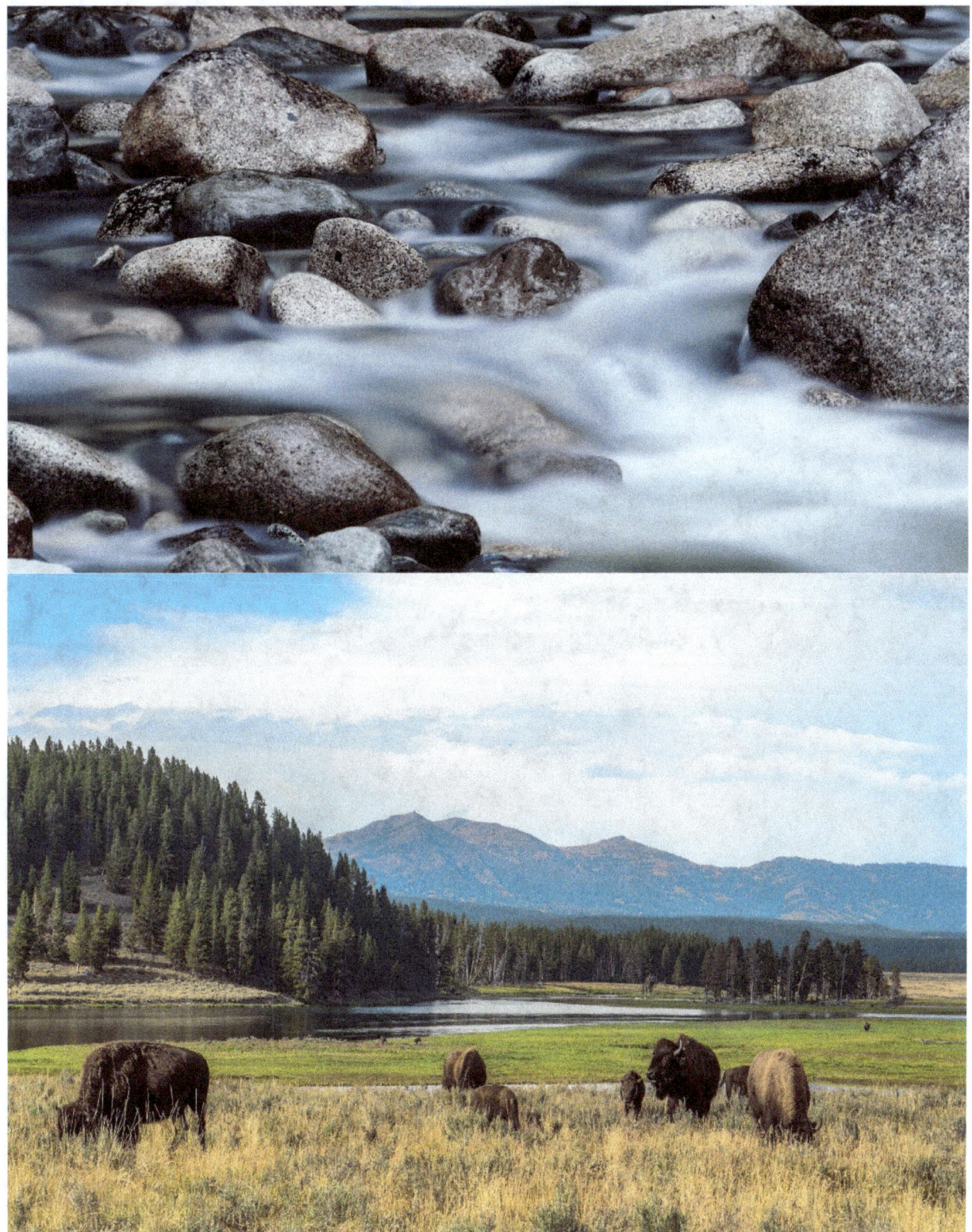

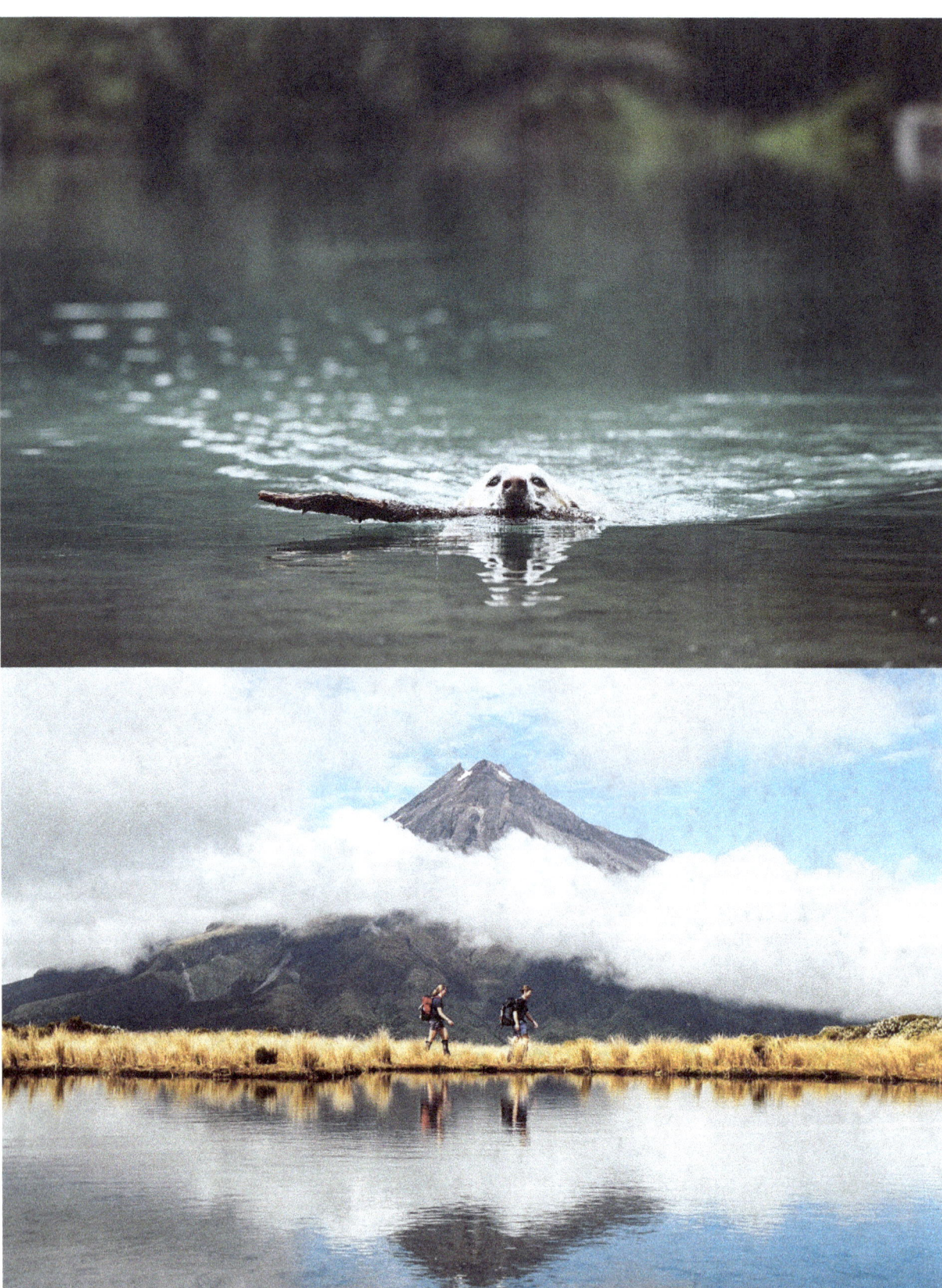

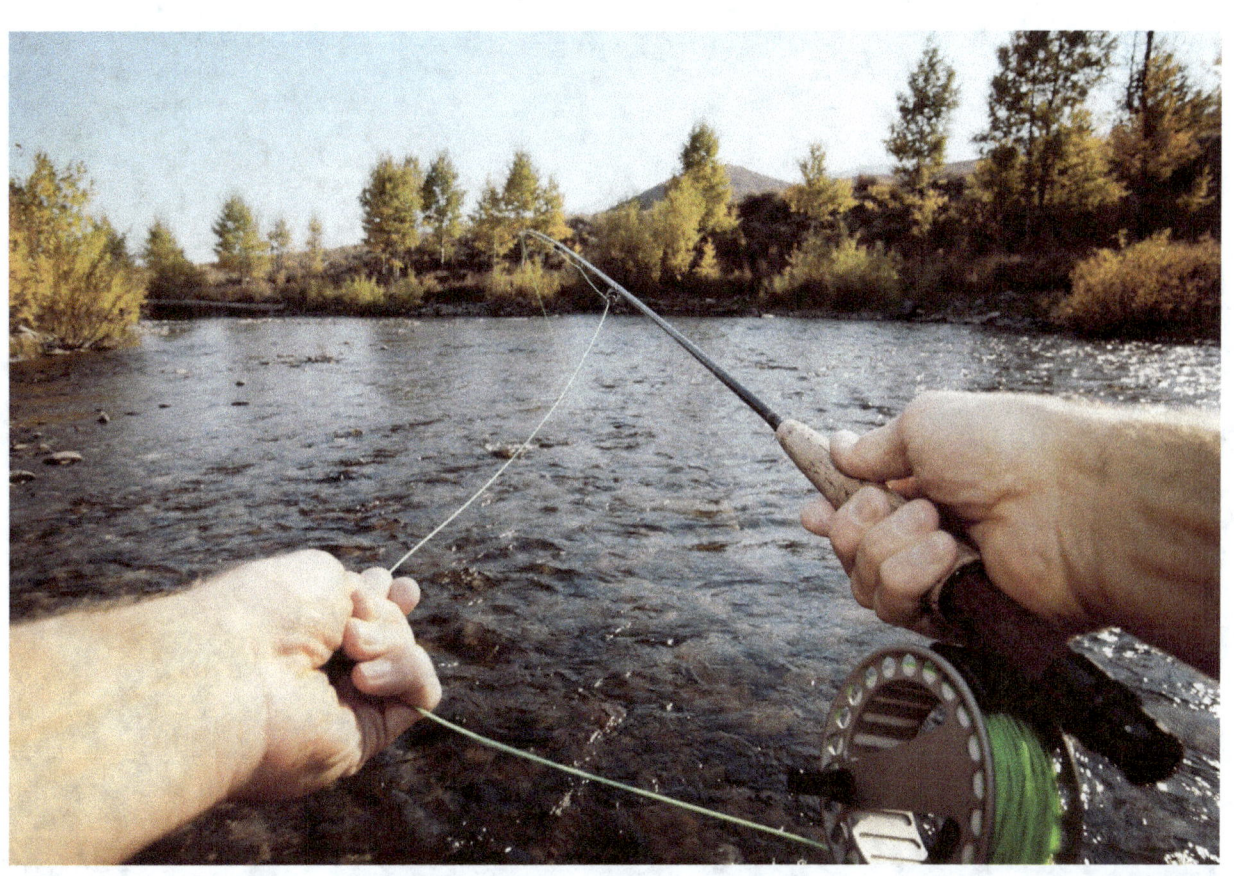

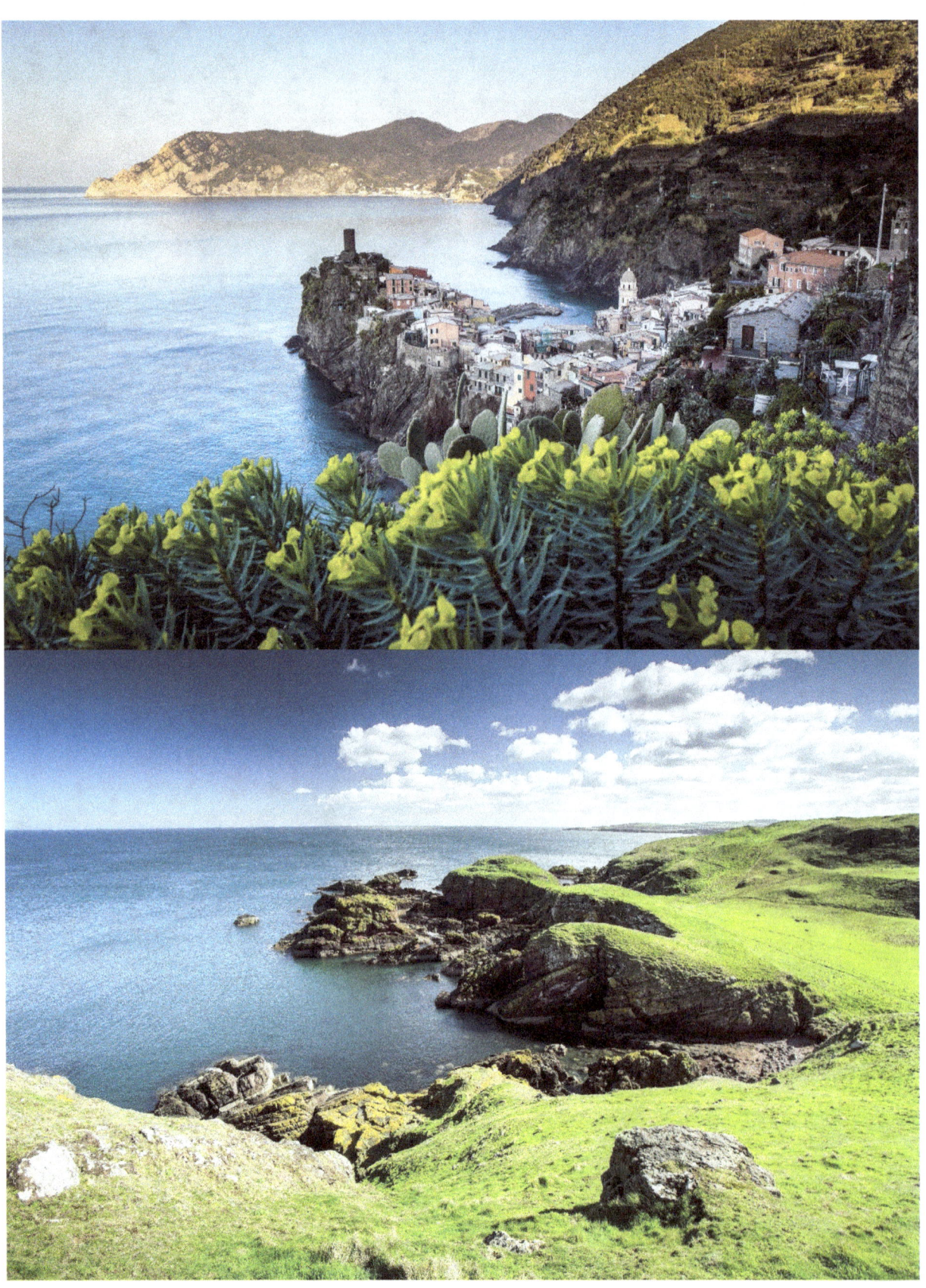

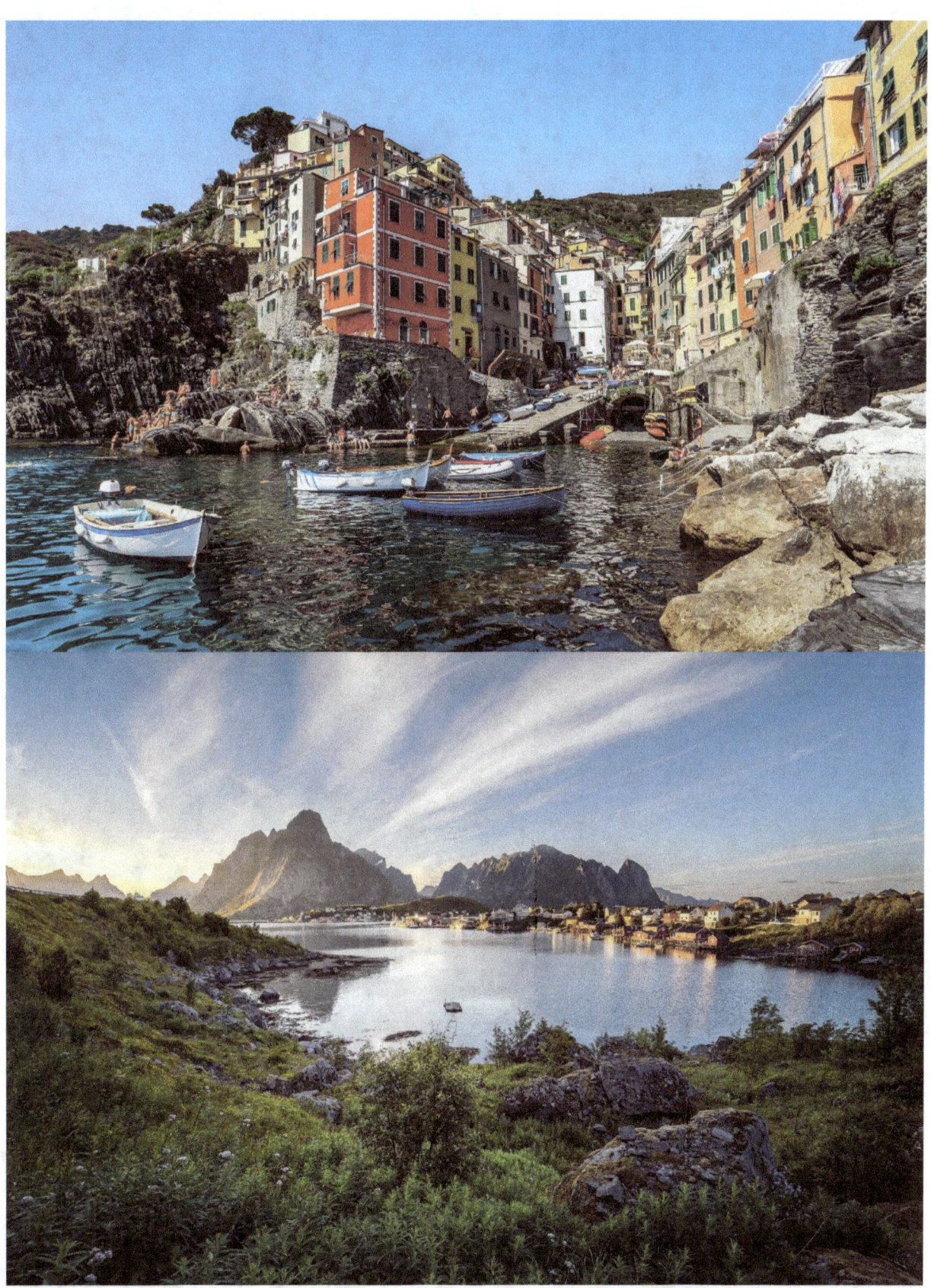

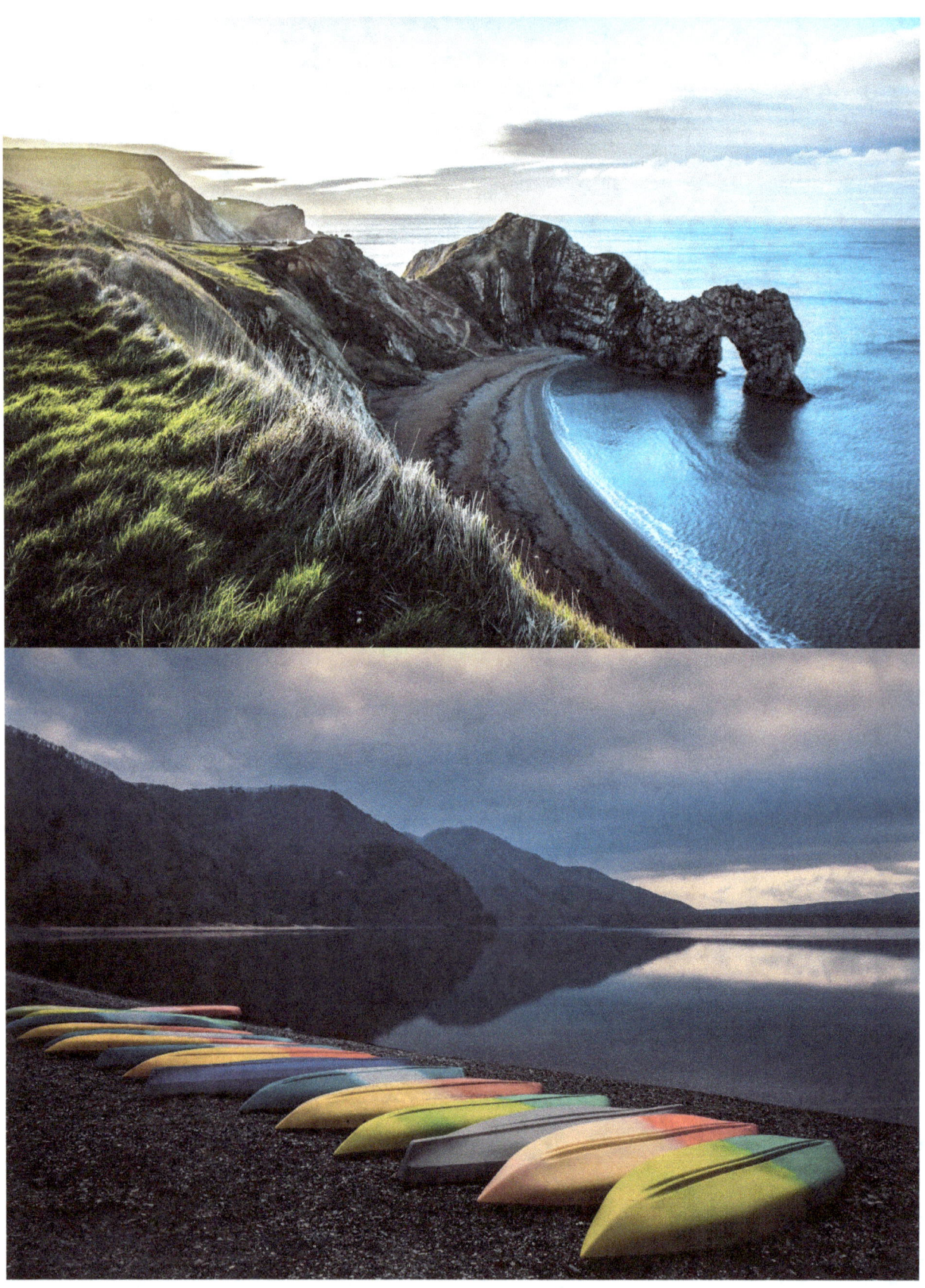

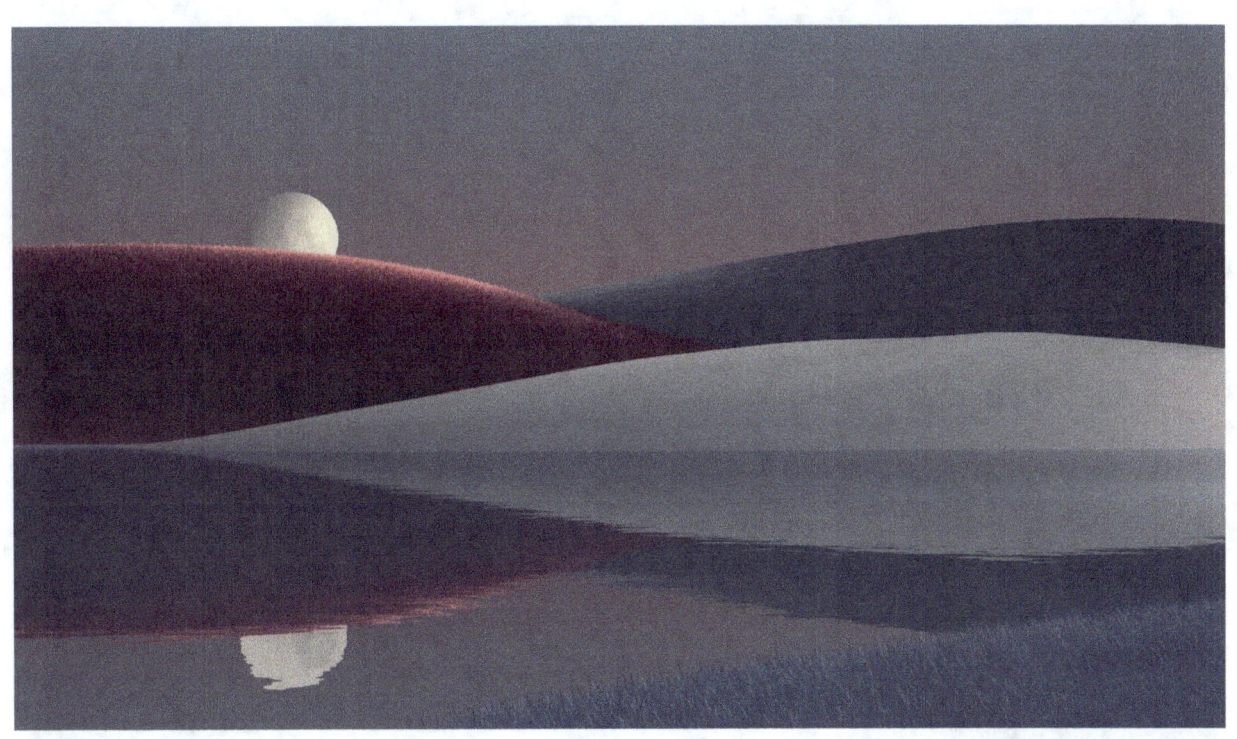

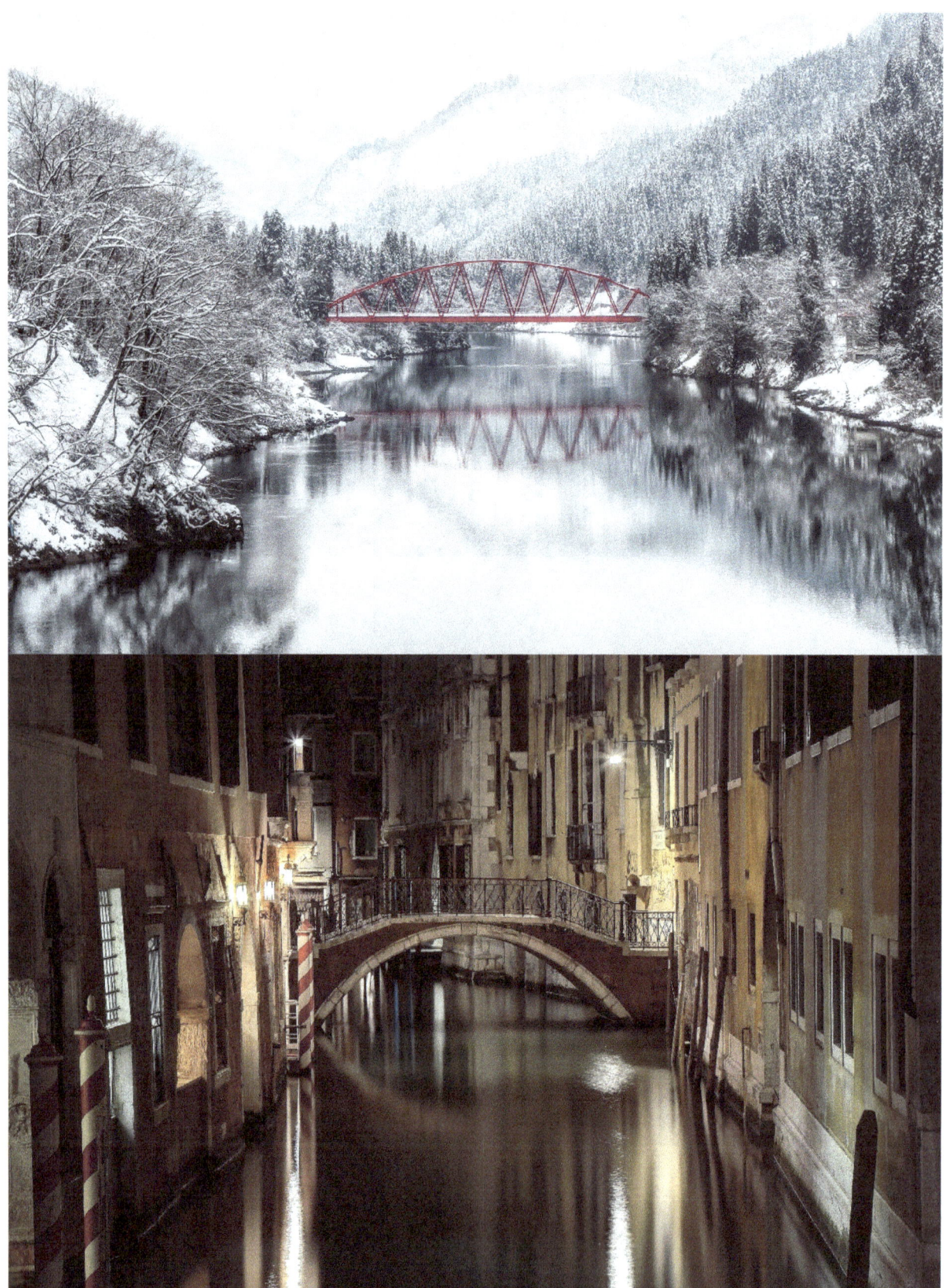

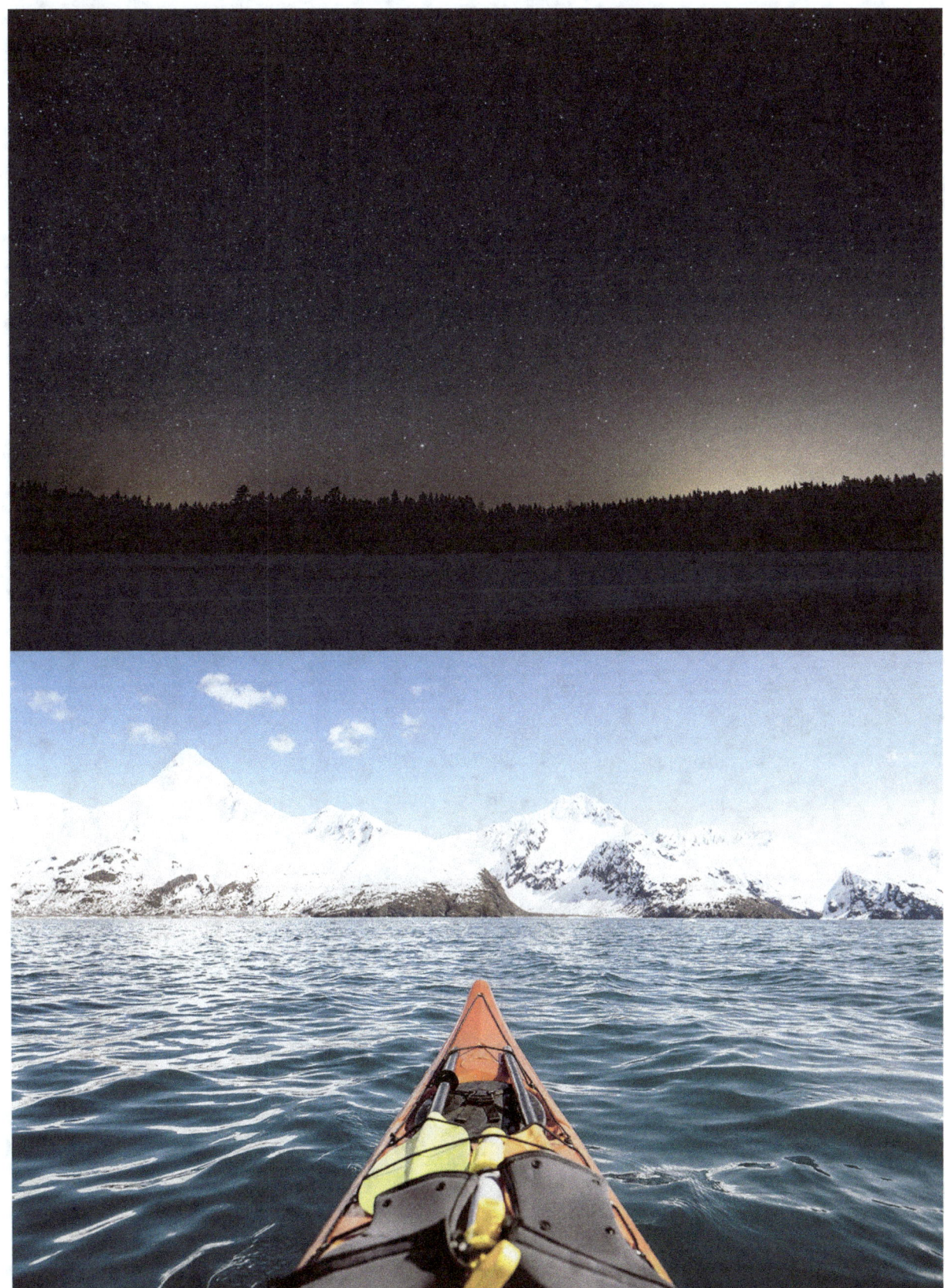

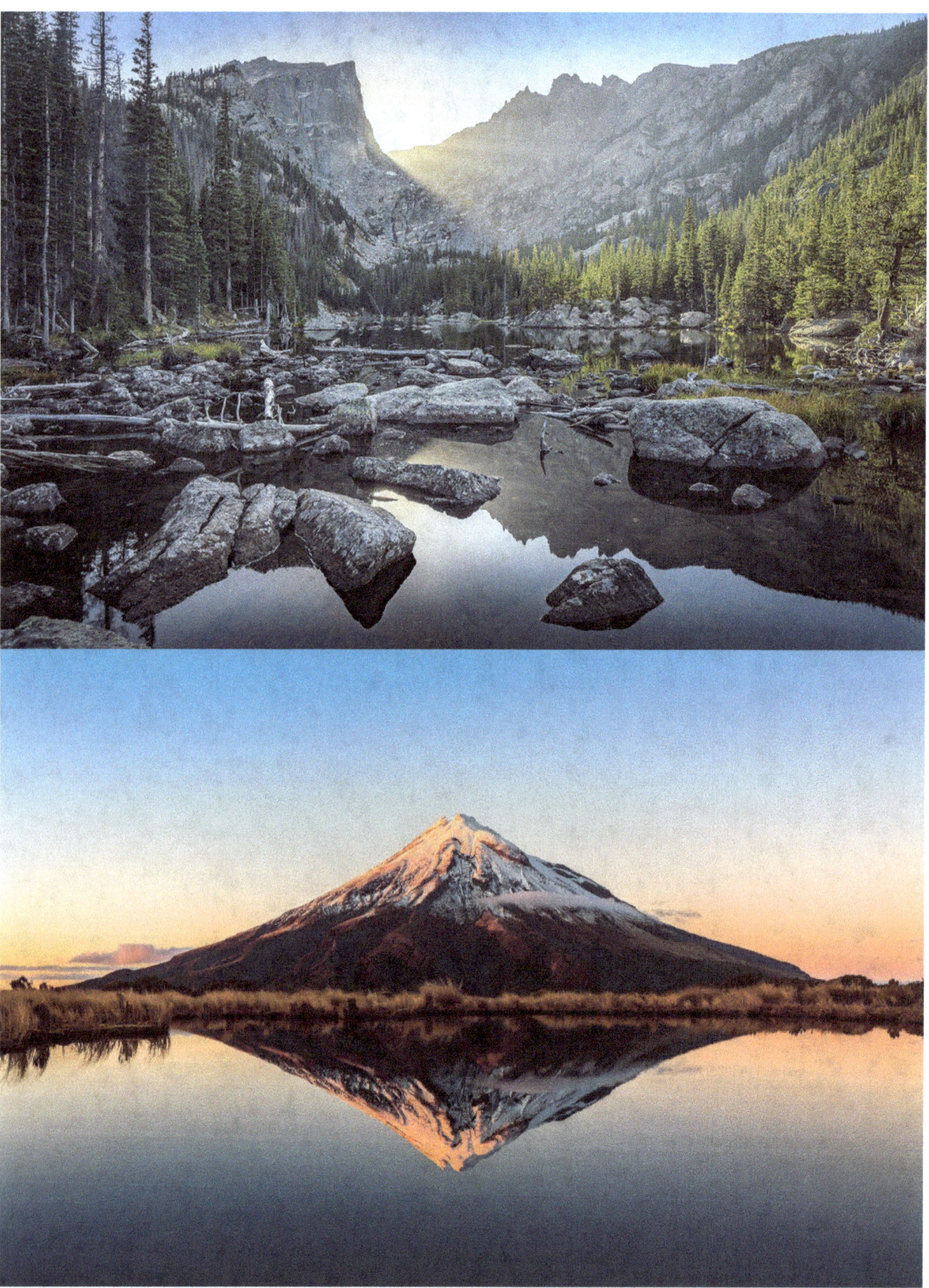

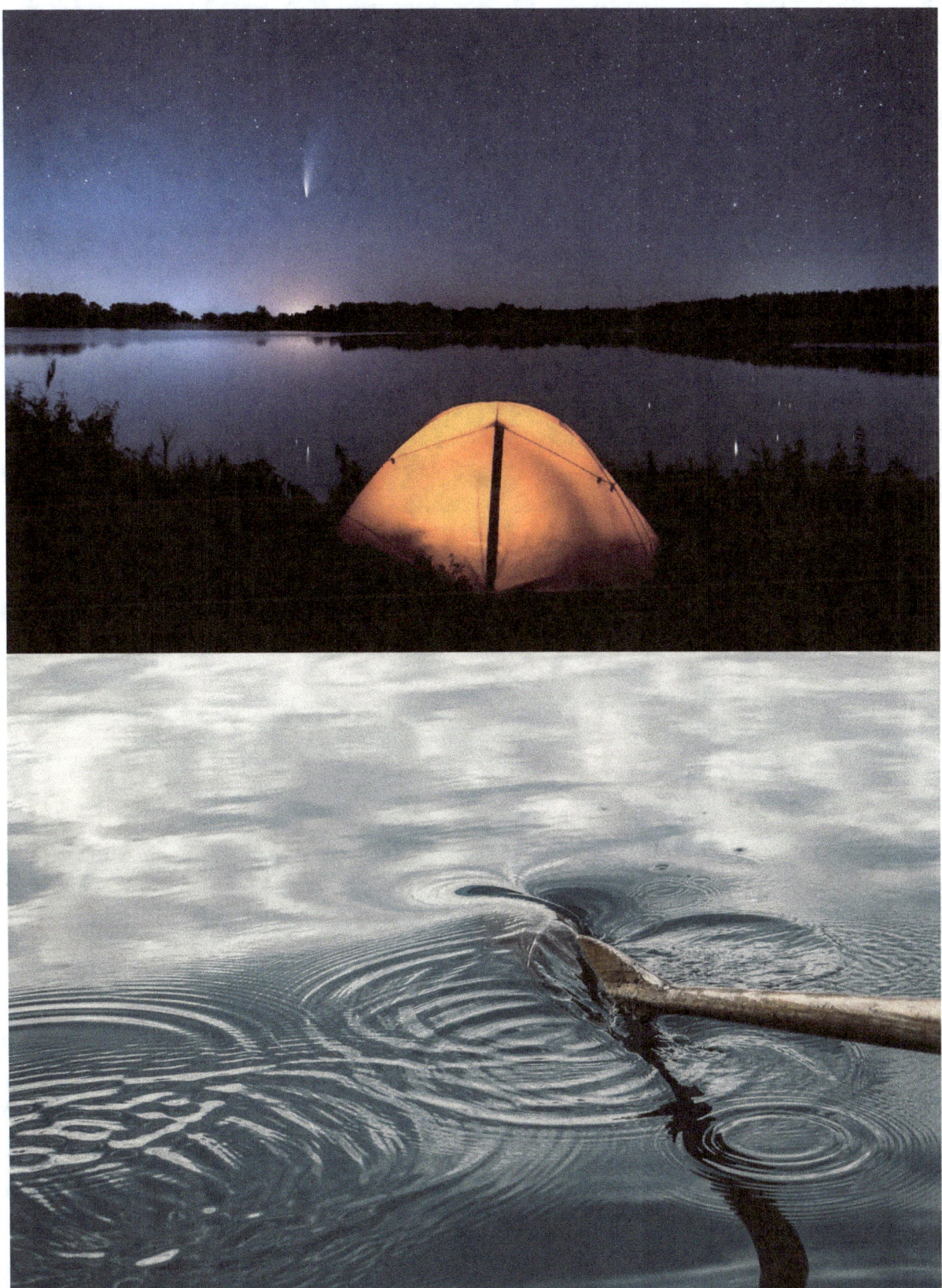

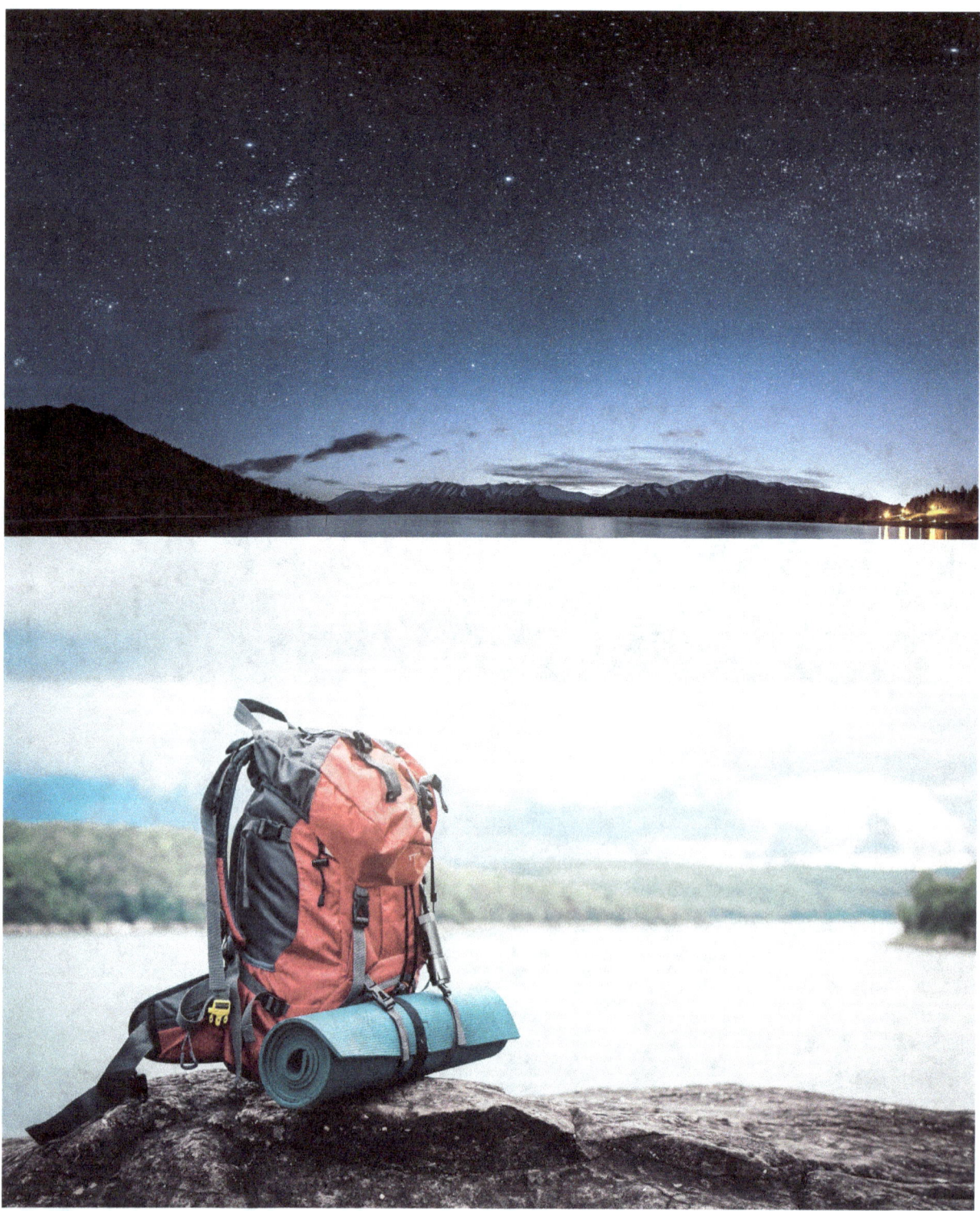

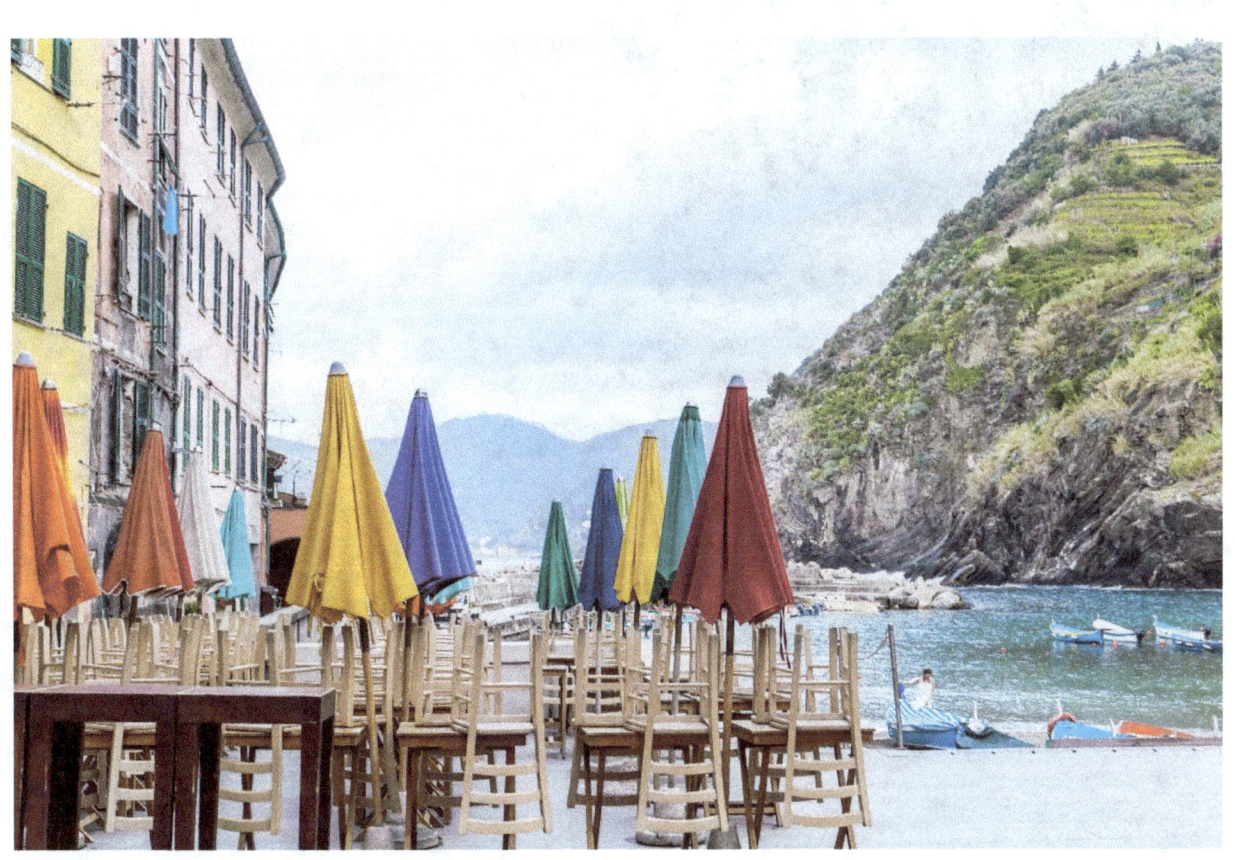

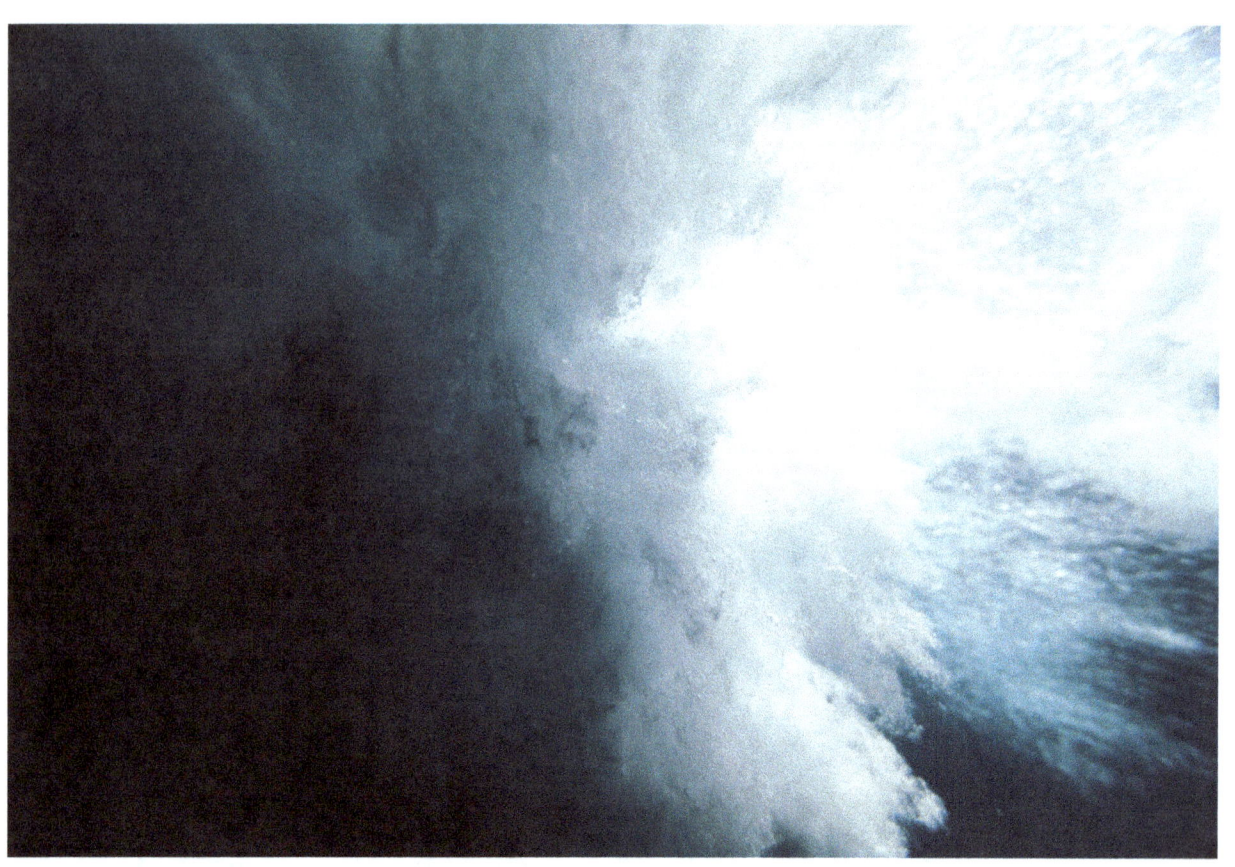

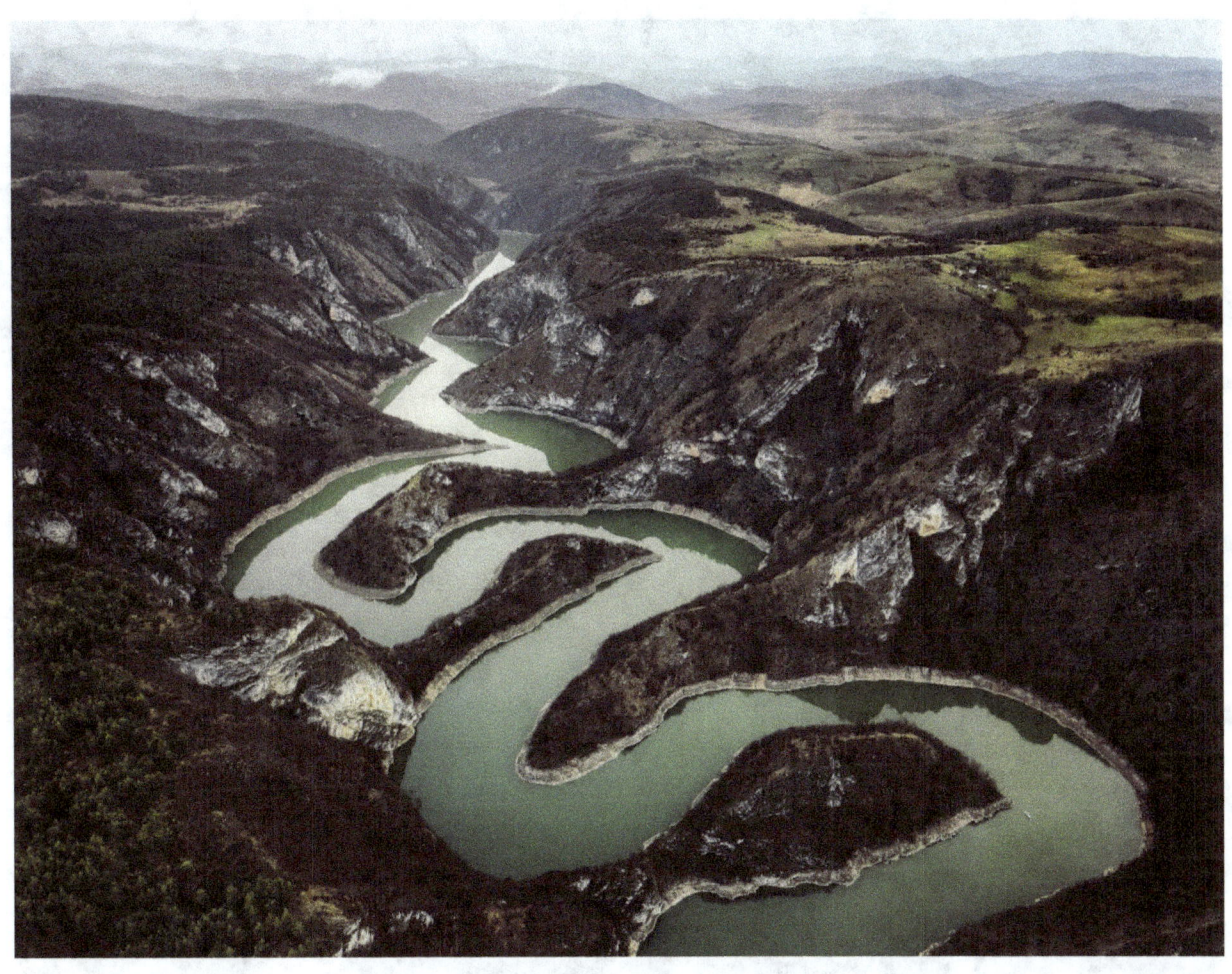

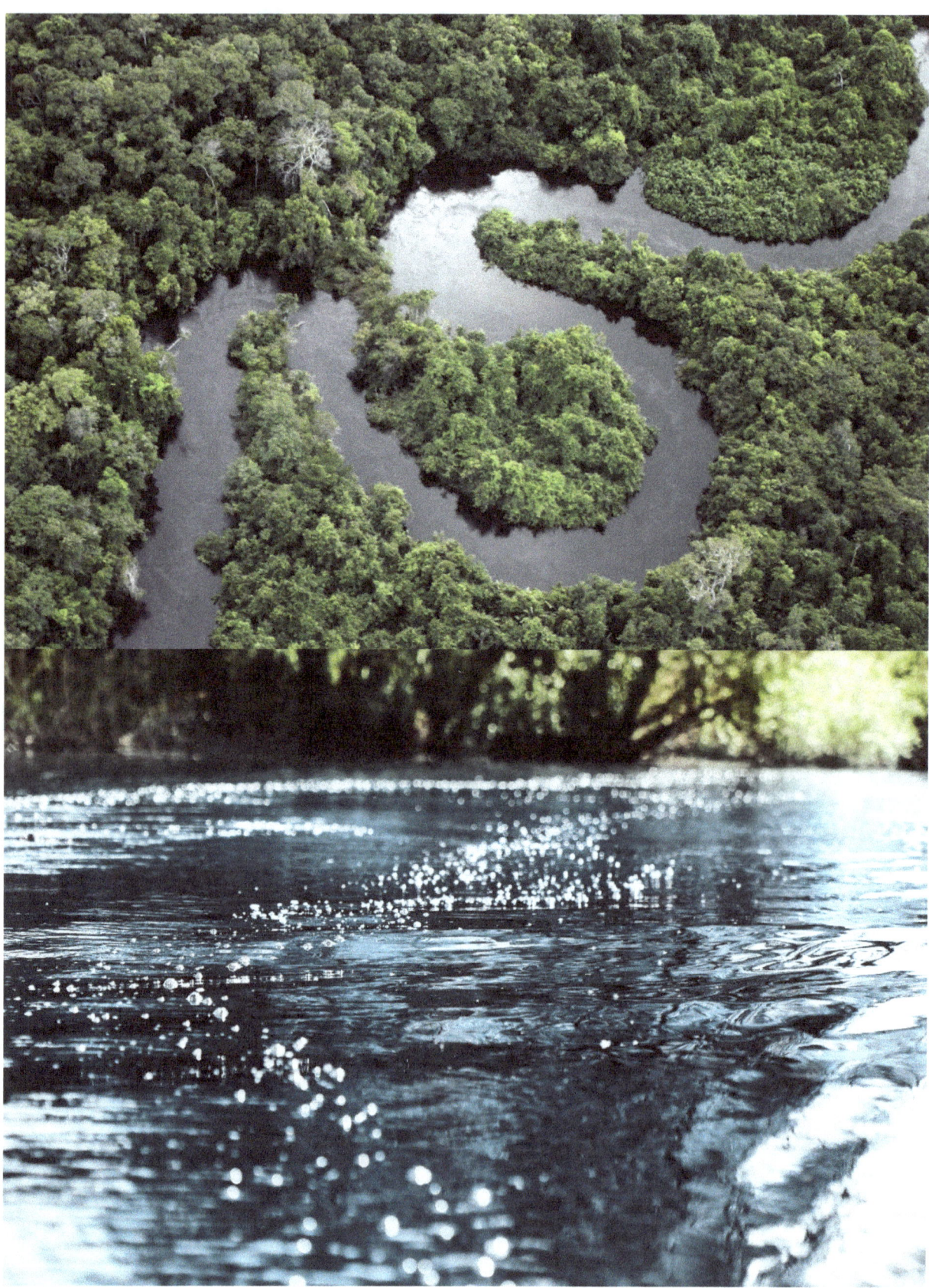

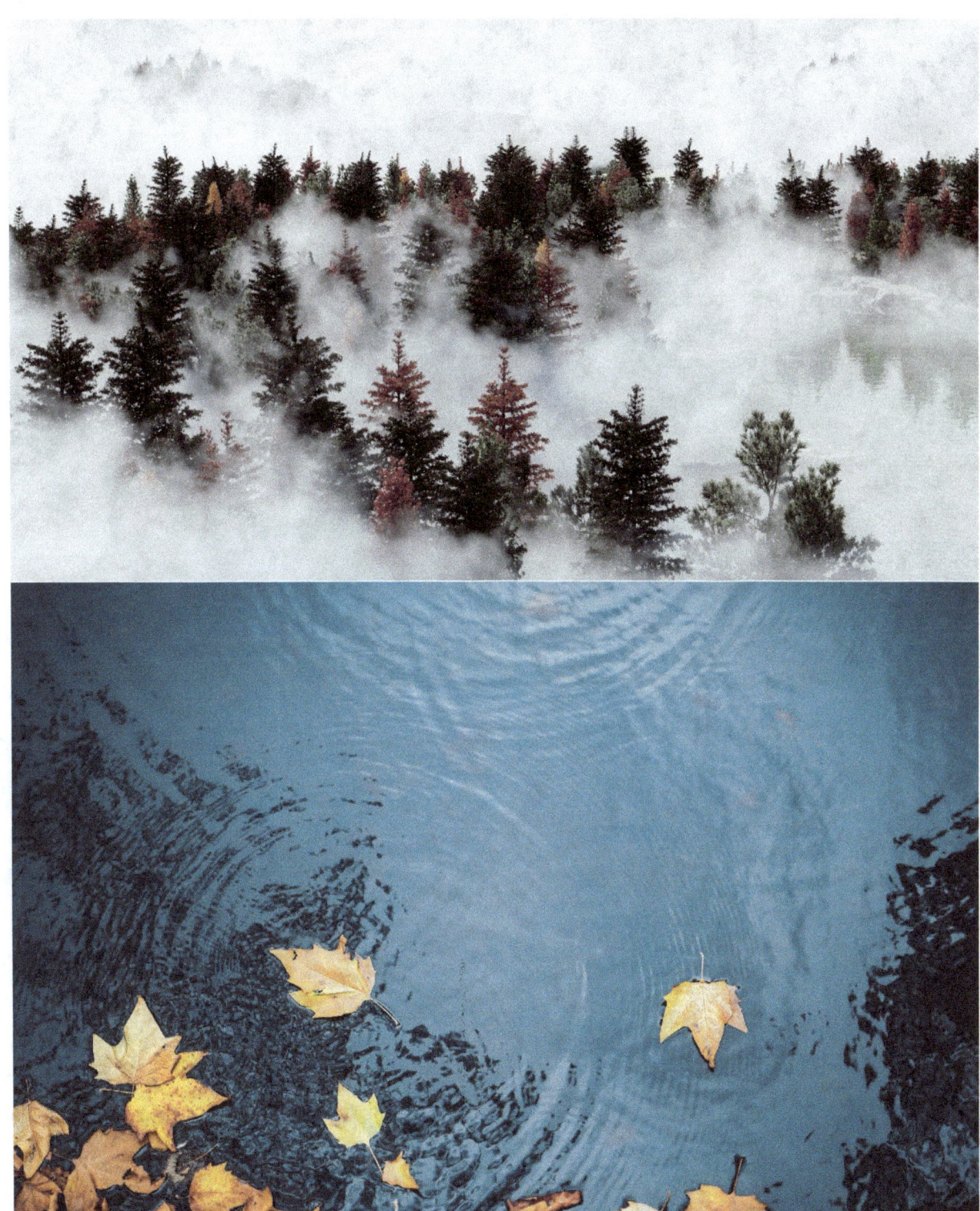

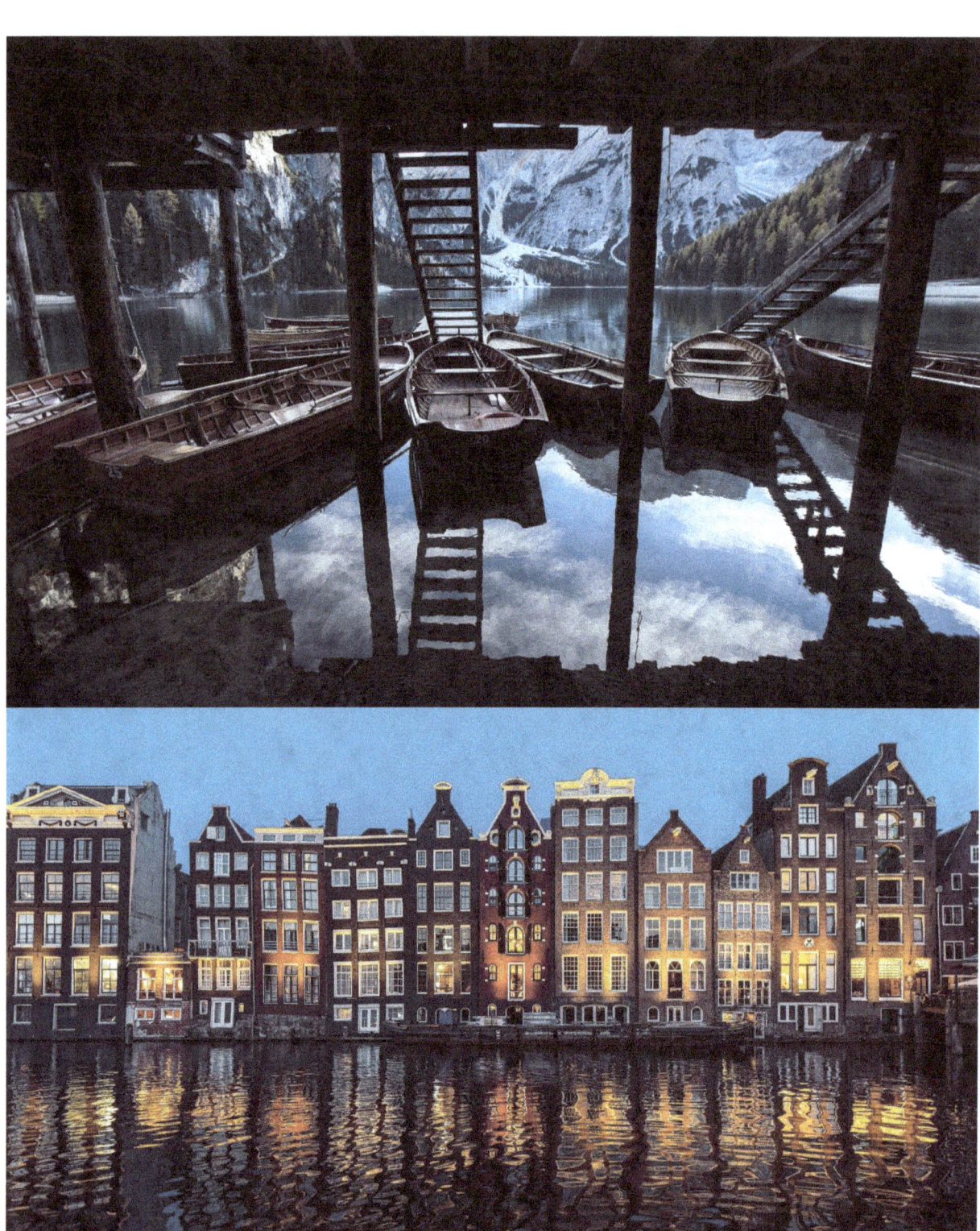

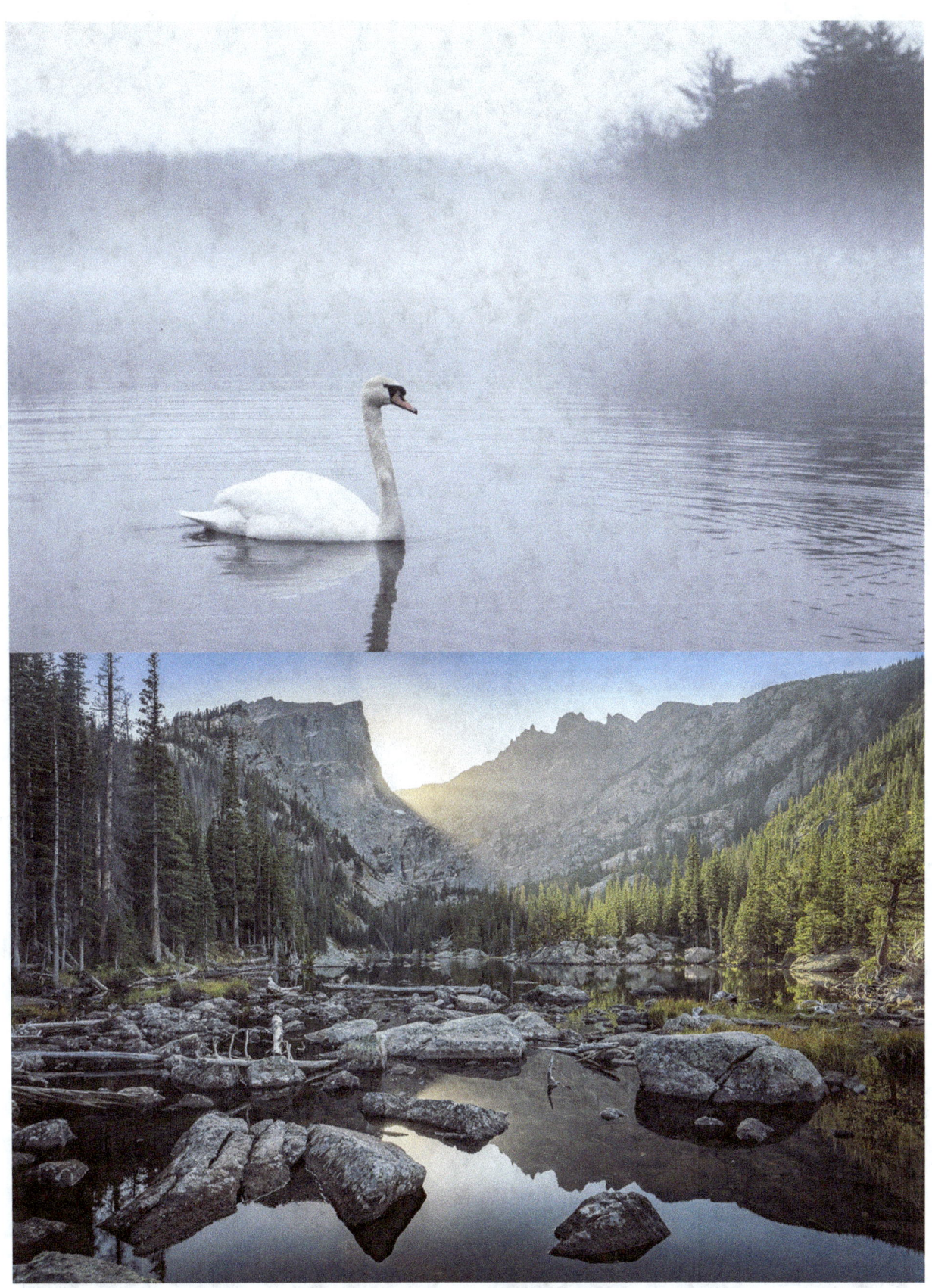

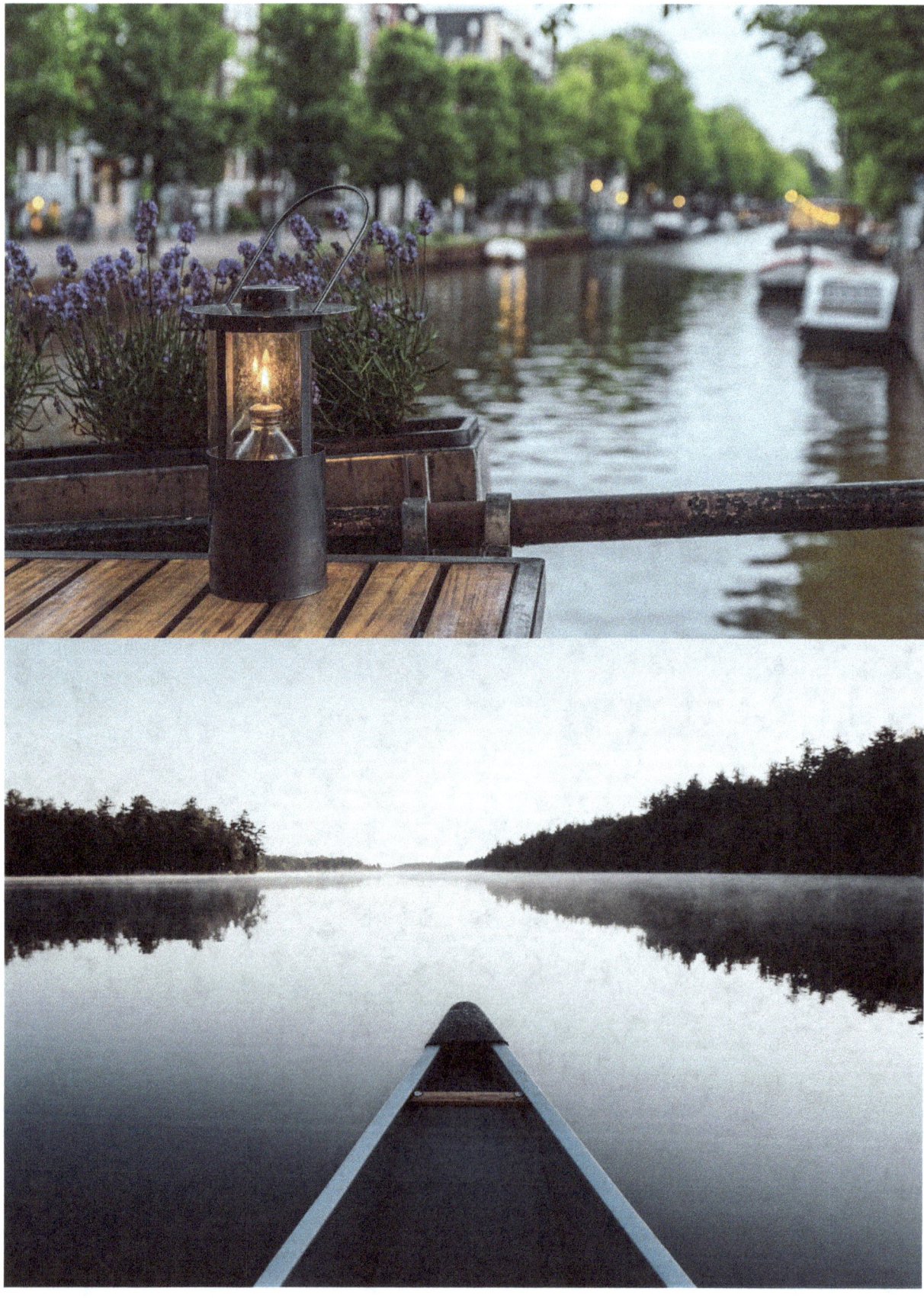

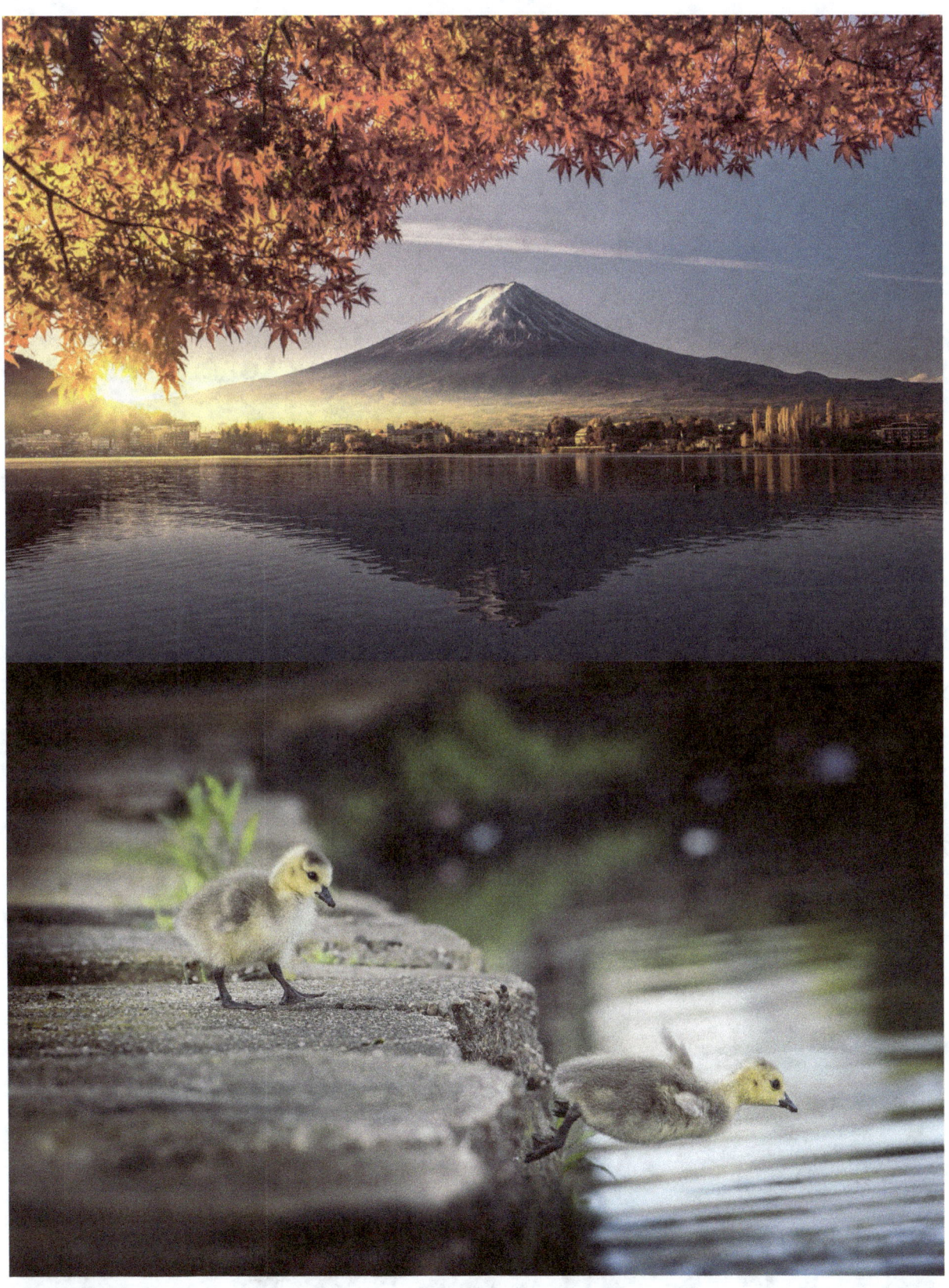

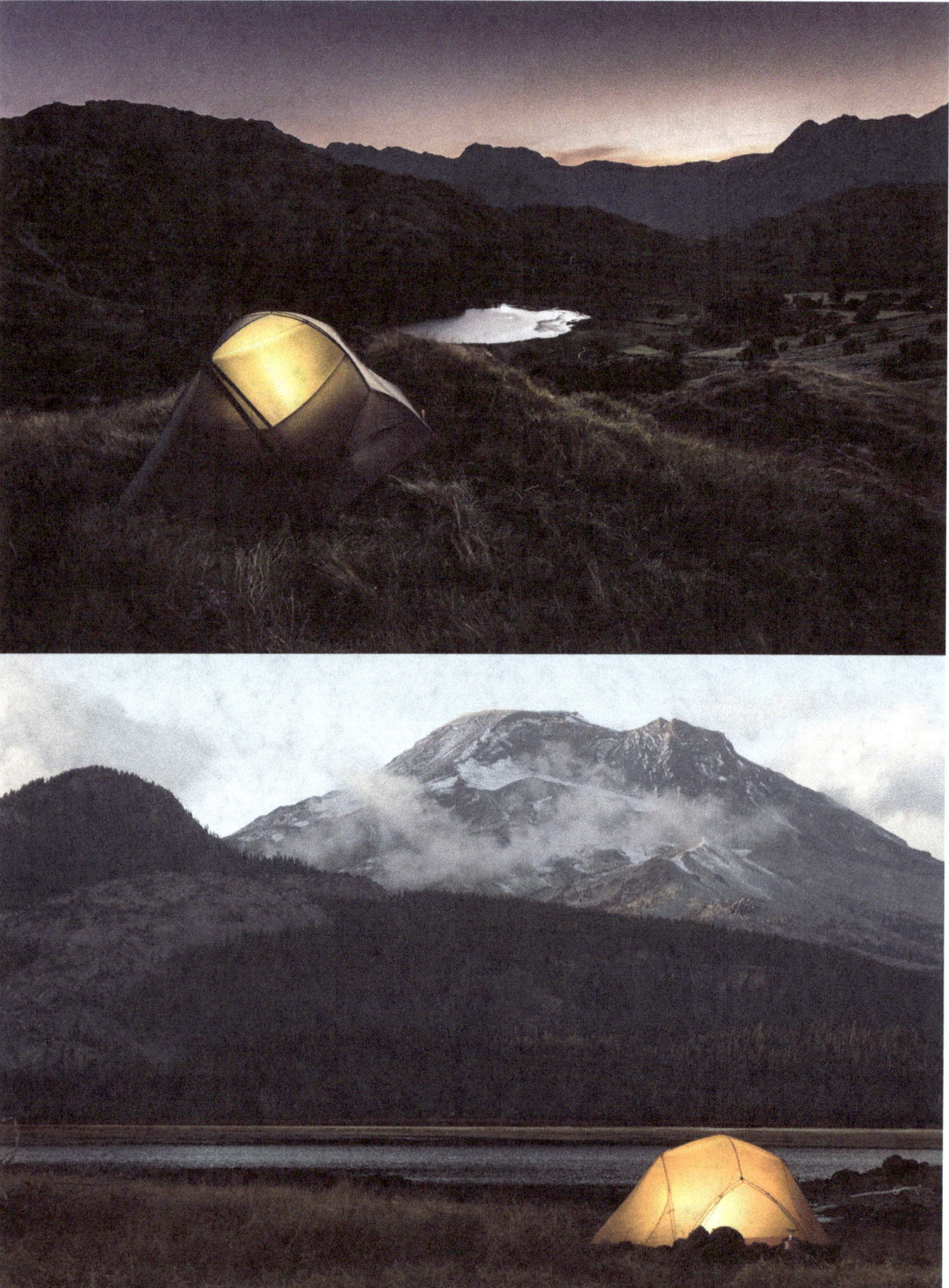

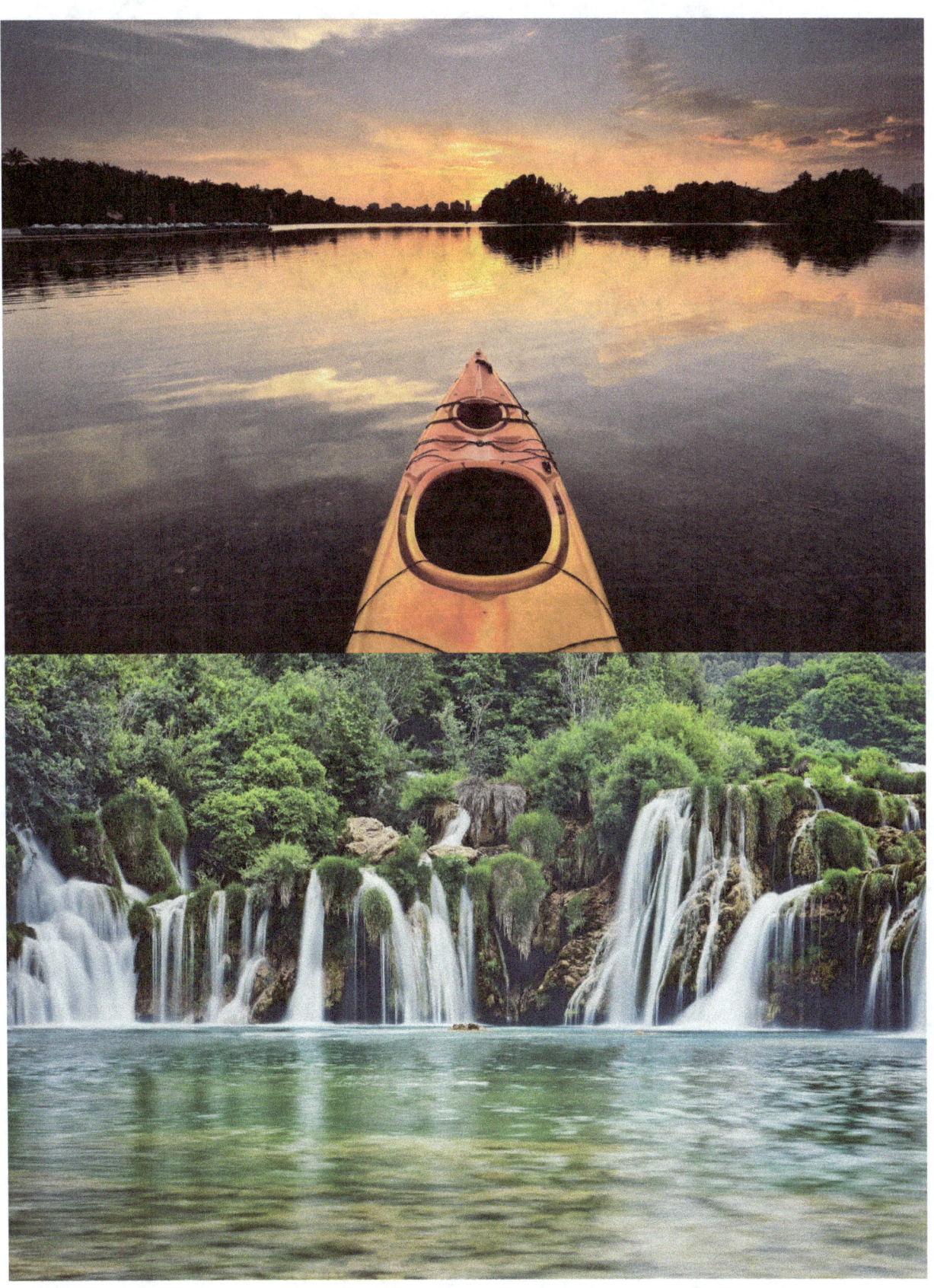

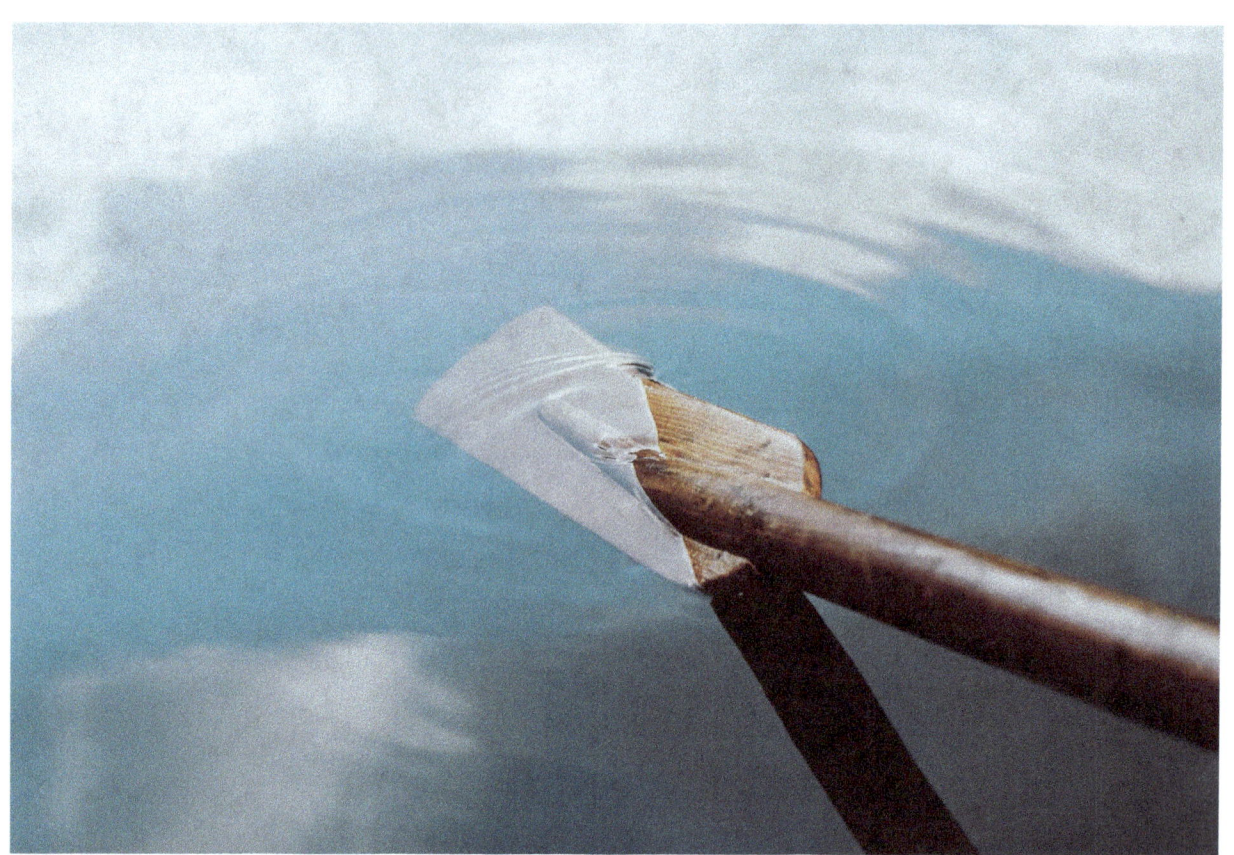

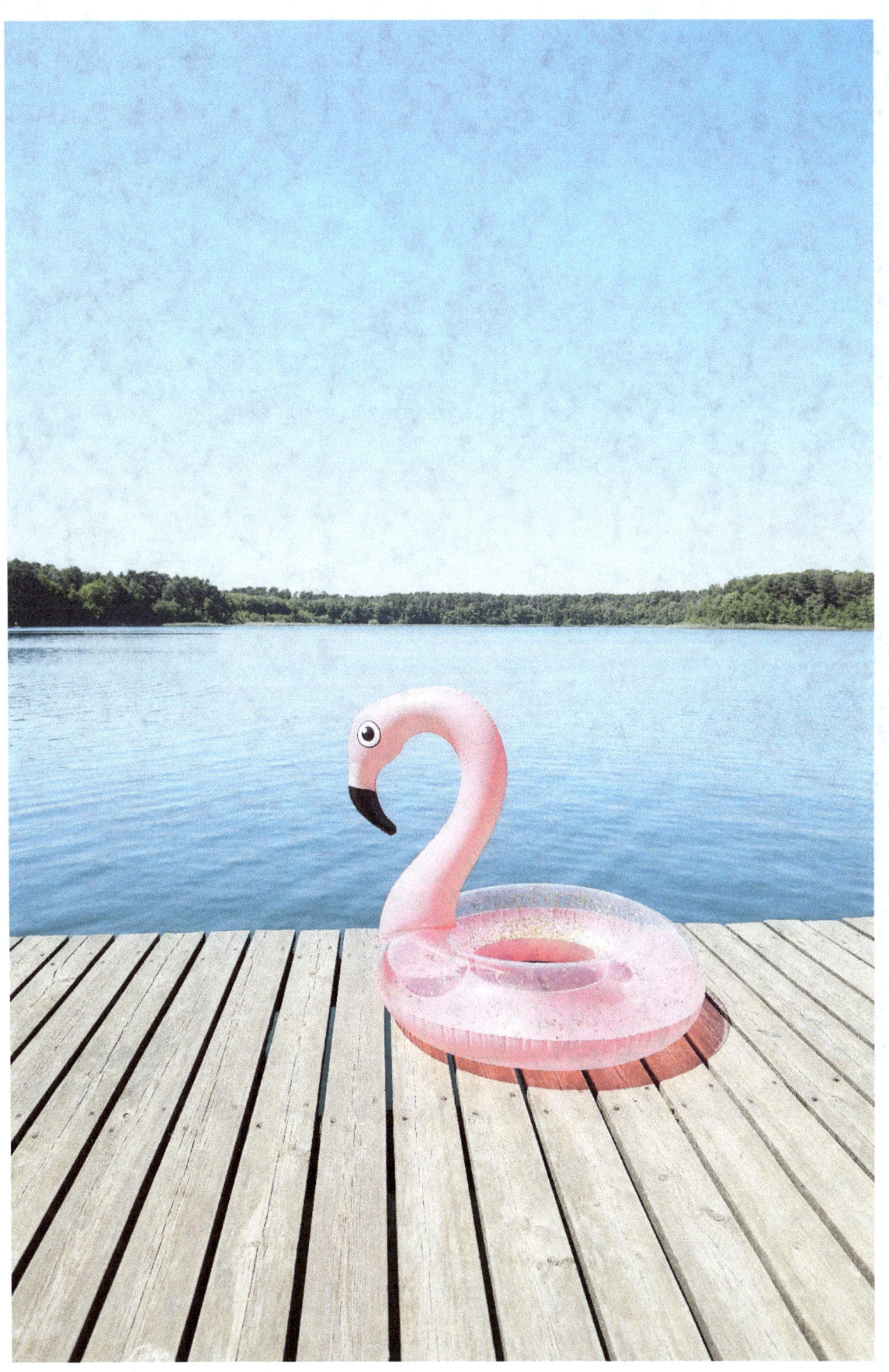

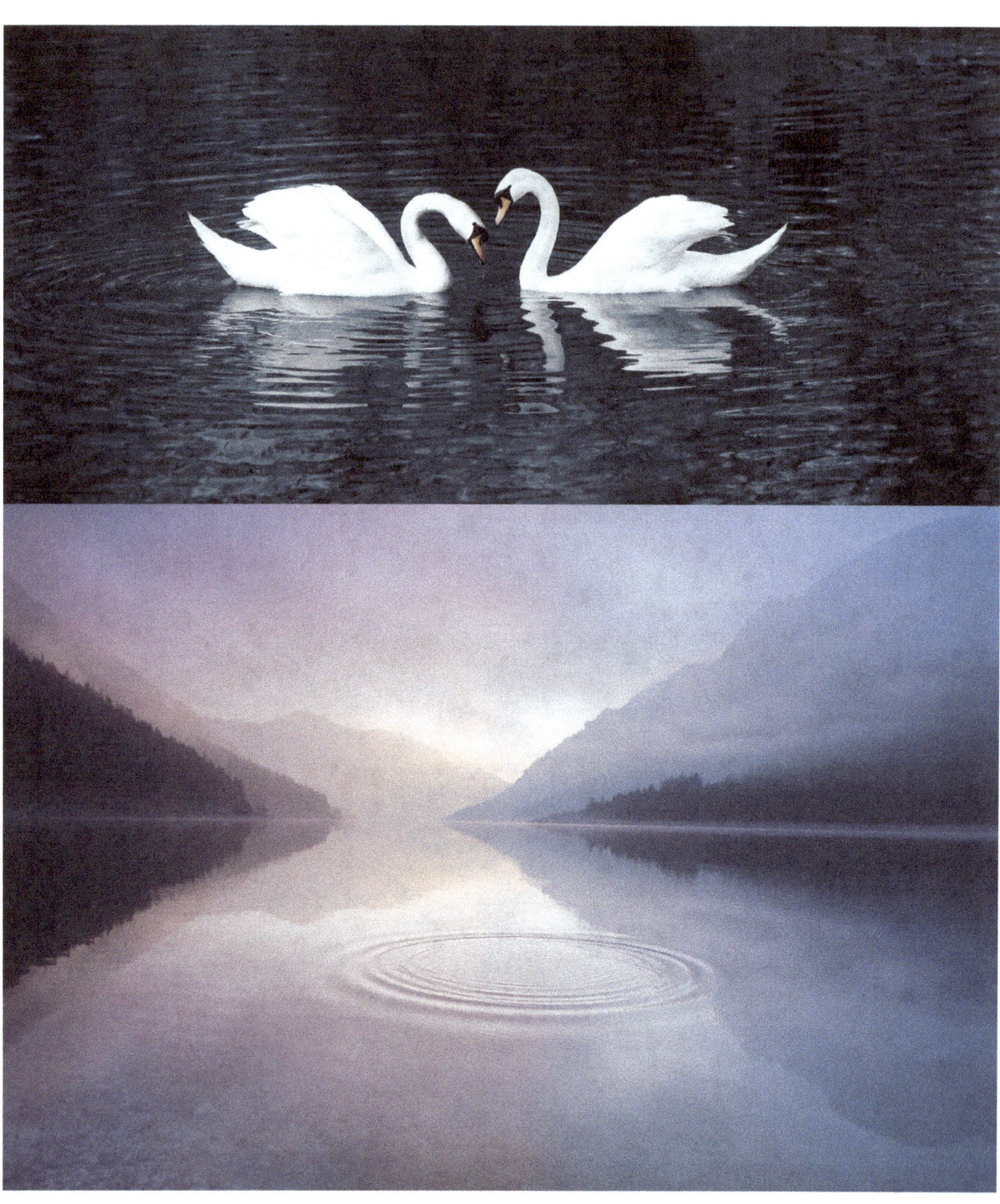

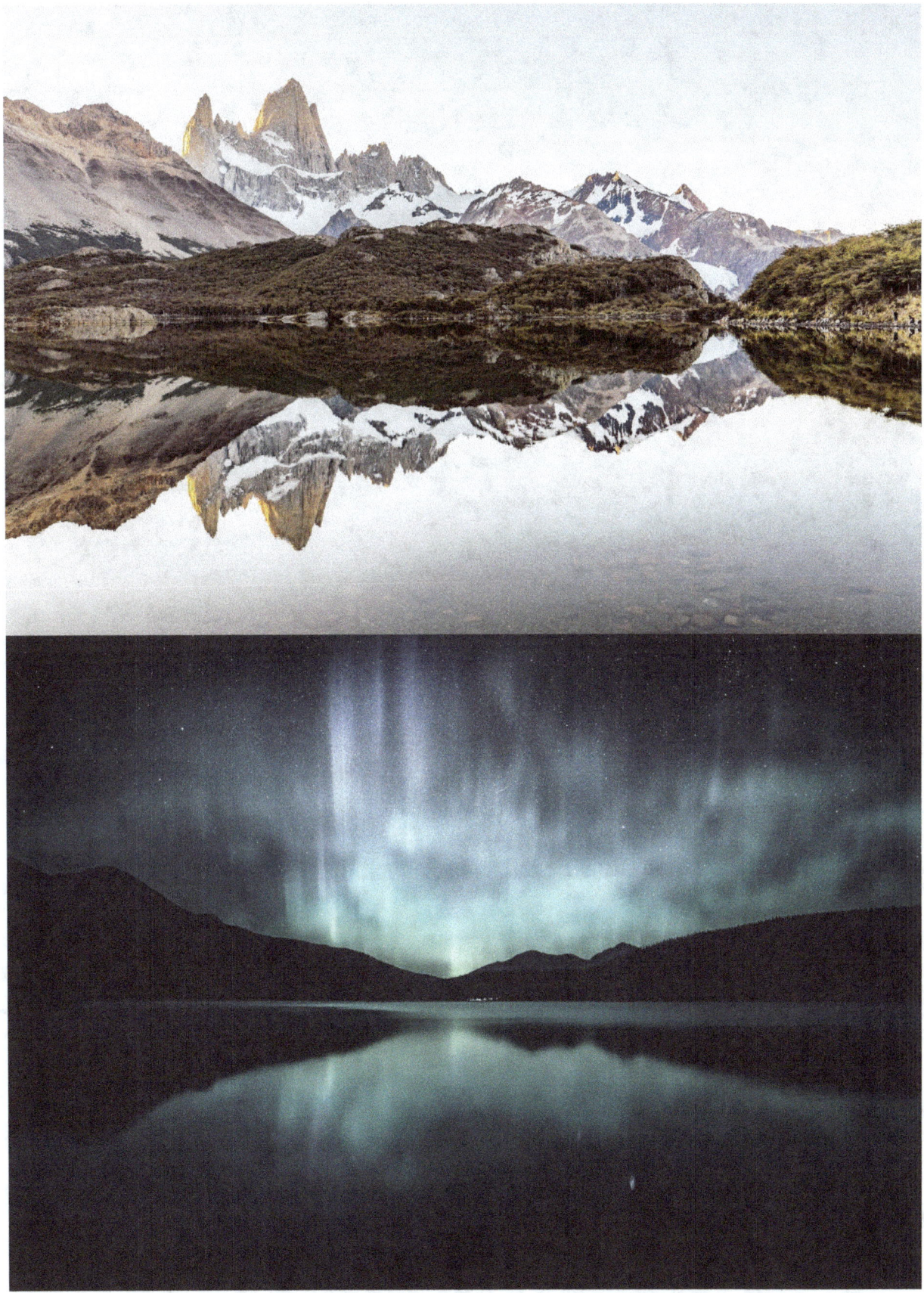

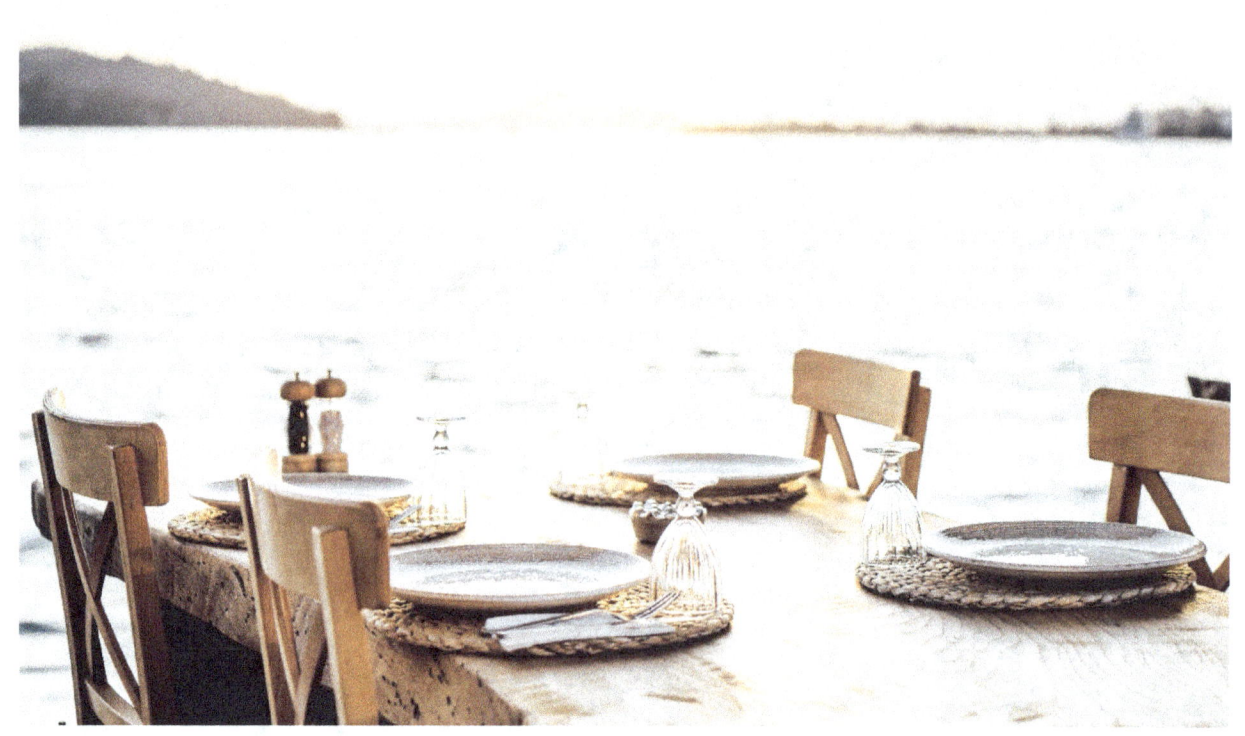

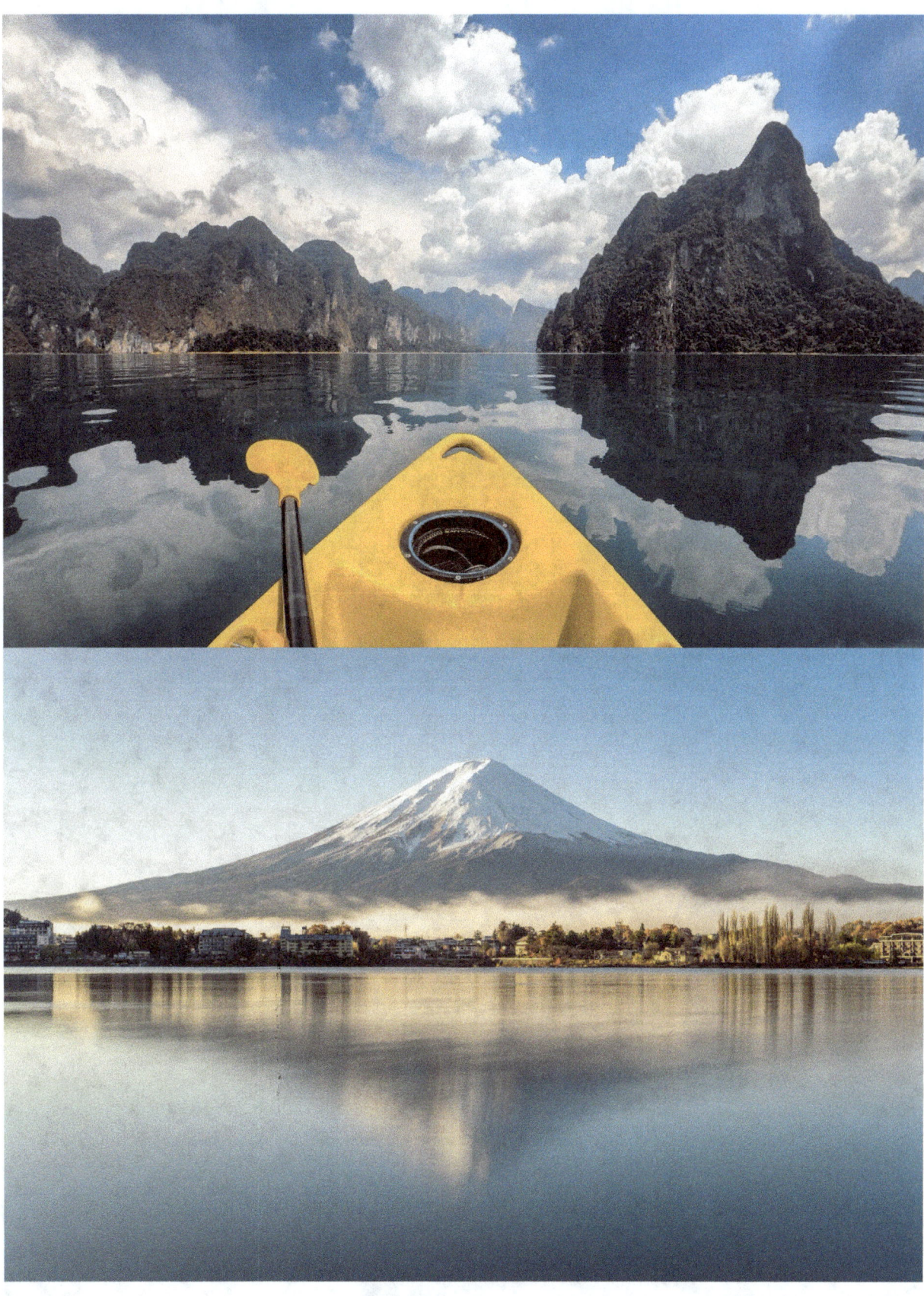

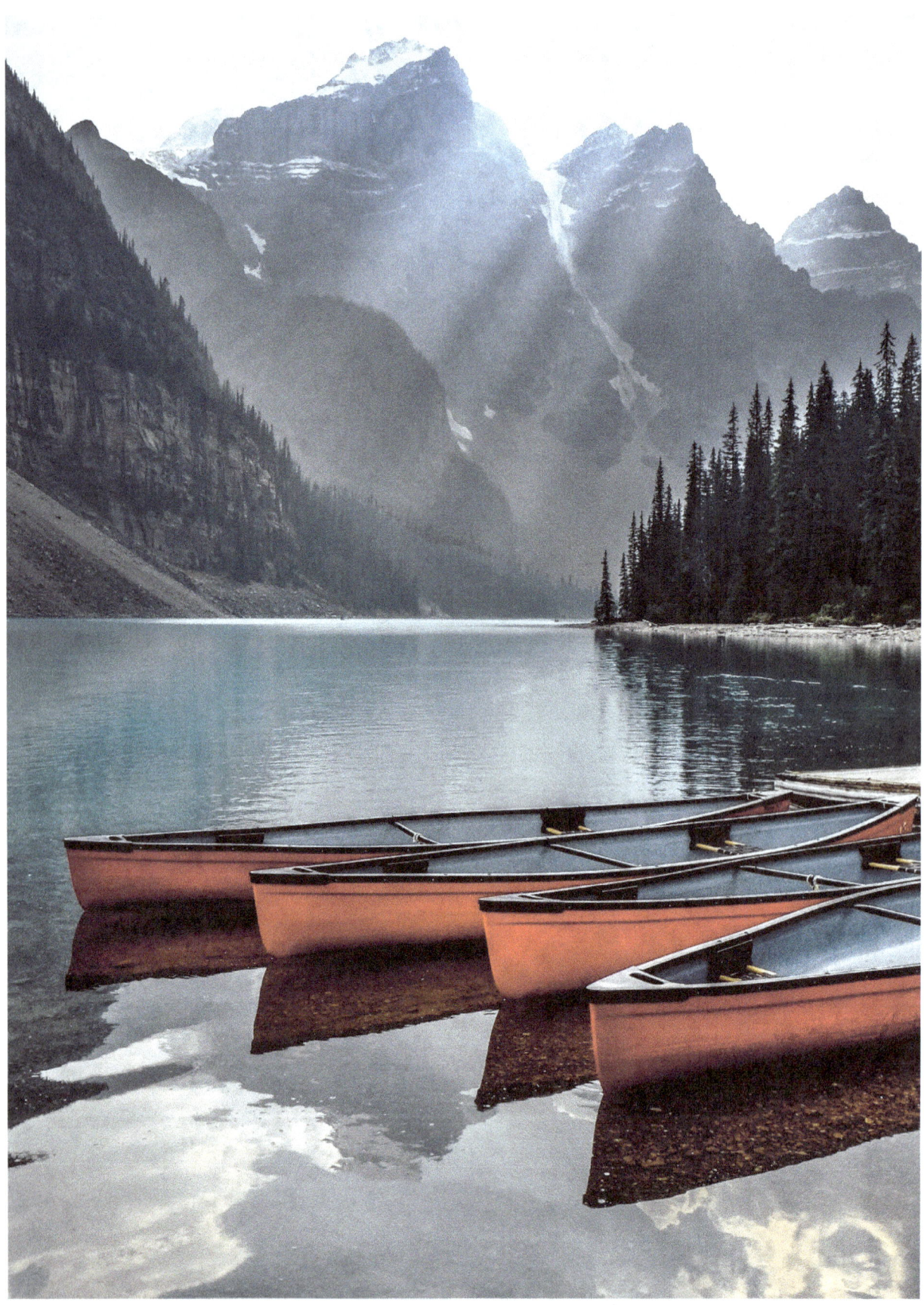

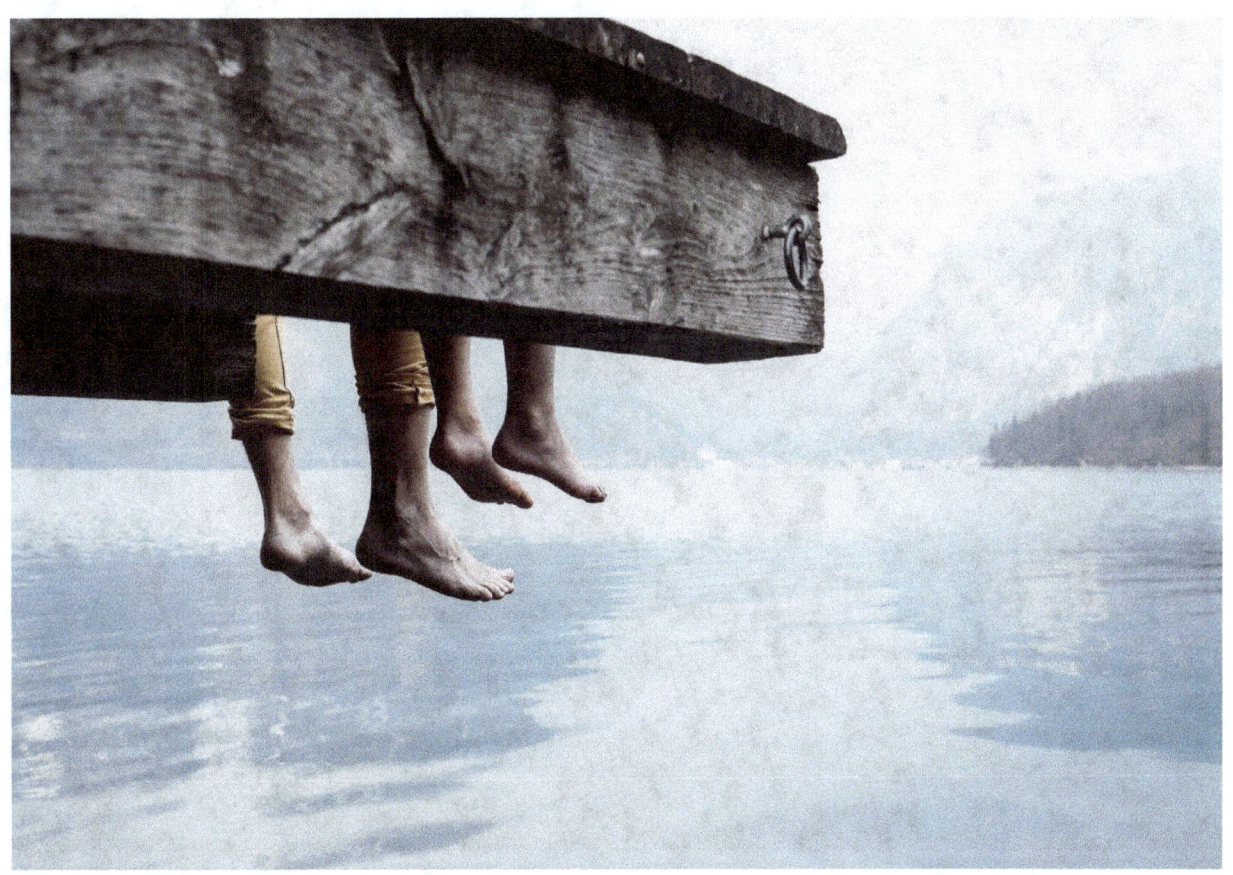

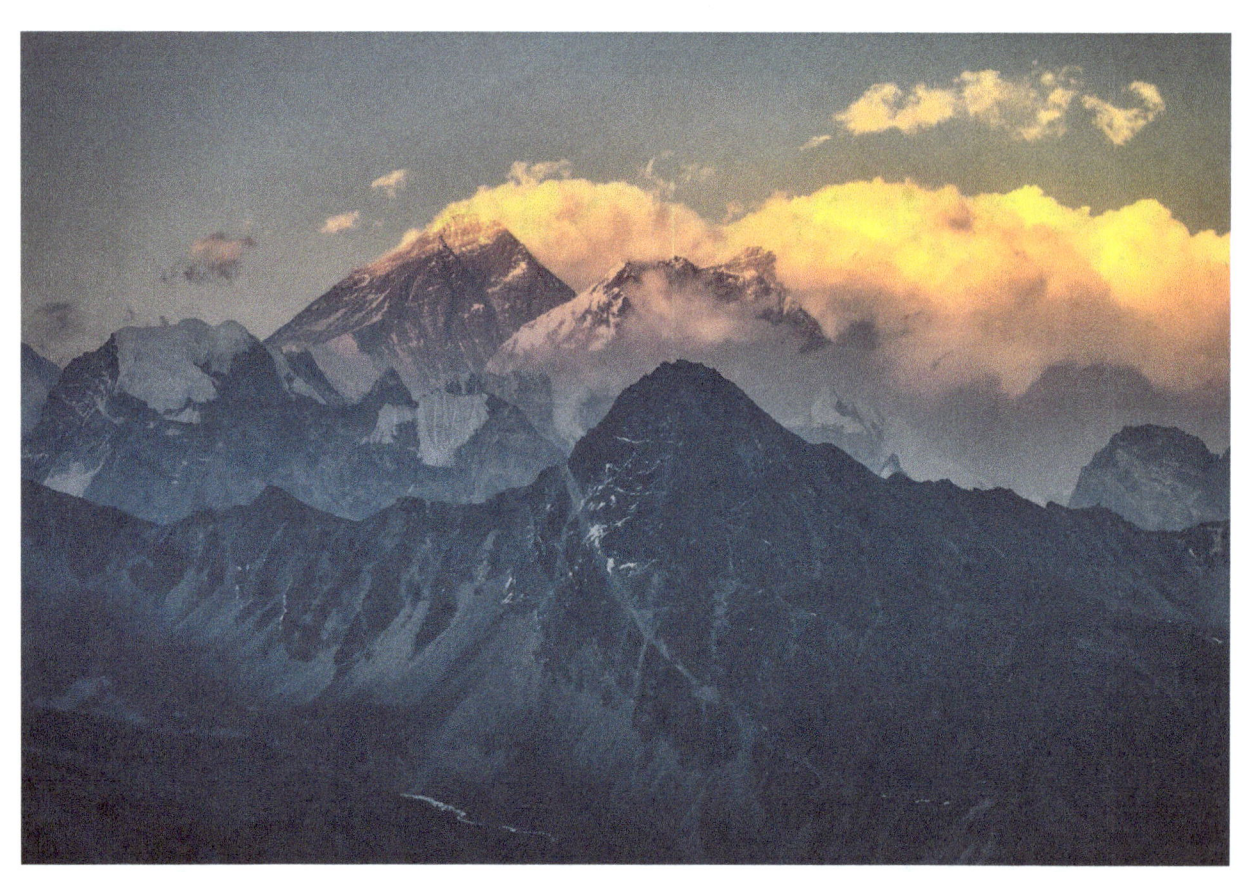

The End

In Loving Memory of Zan

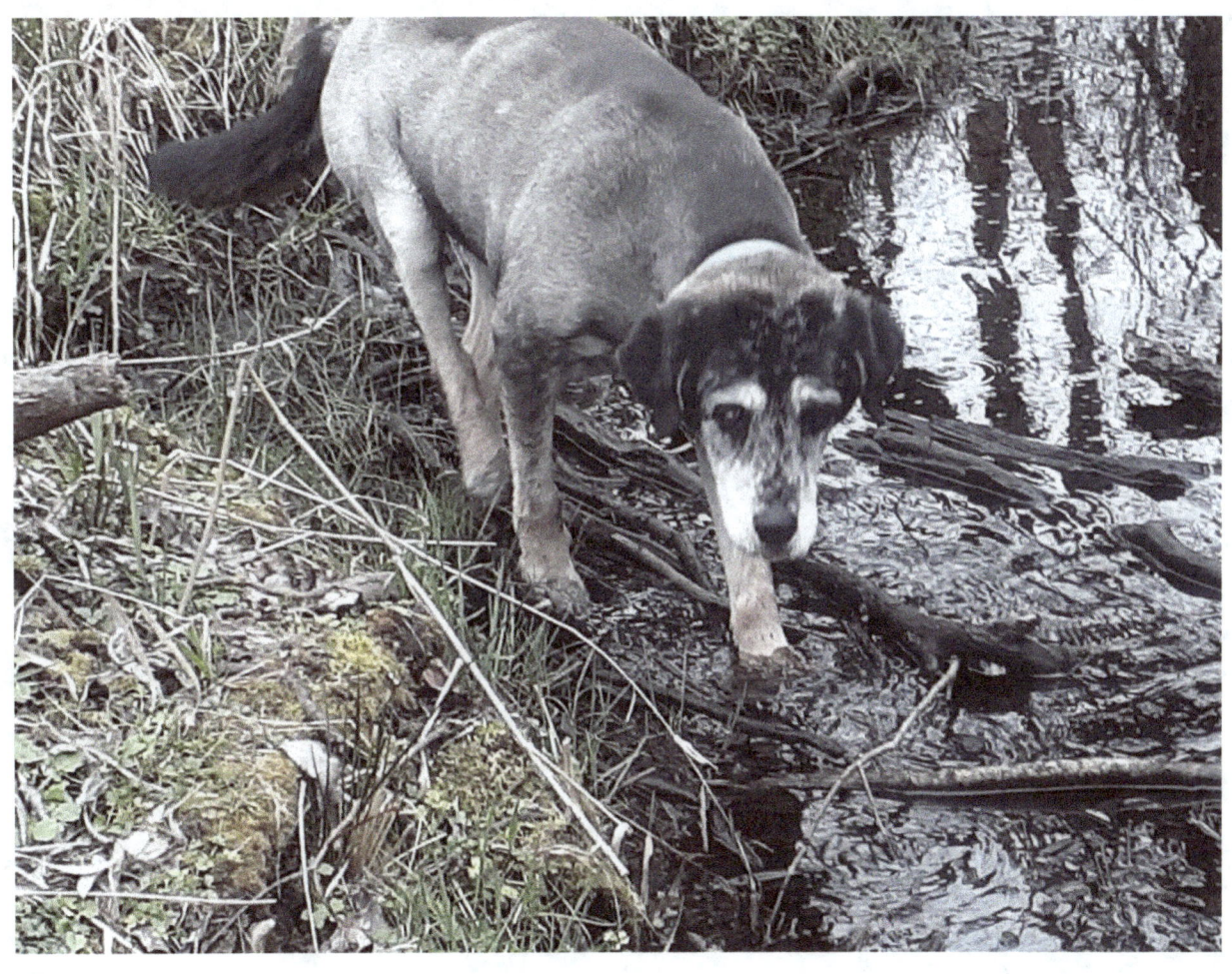

March 11, 2022